Sex Positions

Three Book Bundle Including BDSM Roleplays & Sub/Dom Guides

3 books in 1!

BDSM Playbook - The Secret Guide to Being the Submissive

BDSM Playbook - The Secret Guide to Being the Dominant

Marriage Games- Turn Your Bedroom Into A BDSM Dungeon

By: More Sex More Fun Book Club

Hey,

Thank you very much for choosing this book!

Before we begin...

If you are interested in non-fiction sex books, head over to our partner site alexandramorris.com

Alexandramorris.com is a great site in the making. They publish e-books, paperbacks, audiobooks and blog posts written by up-and-coming writers and great freelancers. They also give away TONS of Audible coupon codes, Amazon gift cards, pdf copies of books totally free!

We really hope this books will give you valuable information to take your sex life to the next level. Enjoy and please leave an honest review after finishing it.

Best regards

Table of Contents

BDSM Playbook

The Secret Guide to Being the Submissive

Introduction

This book contains proven information on how to clearly define the parameters and traits of a submissive, how to identify true submissive traits within yourself, and what roles a submissive can take on within the BDSM and Dominant/Submissive paradigms.

In this book, you will find advice and reference points in finding out what a submissive is and whether or not you happen to be one. You will be given a taste on how to take up your role in a BDSM role play scene and how to be a good submissive to your dominant. You will also find references regarding any toys and tools that can be used in your play to heighten pleasure and satisfaction. Lastly, you will find advice on how to handle certain problems in the Dominant/Submissive relationship that will give you an edge in handling the common pitfalls faced by those who engage in the BDSM and D/s lifestyles.

Chapter 1: What Does It Mean to be a Submissive?

BDSM, which is an acronym for Bondage and Discipline, Dominance and Submission (DS, or D/s) Sadism and Masochism (SM), has become much more popular recently with the success of books like *50 Shades of Grey*, which has women dreaming of a dominant male figure to take control of them. Being a submissive or a dominant, however, doesn't have a certain type. Male or female, whatever the sexual orientation, can be the submissive or the dominant in BDSM role plays. Although scientific studies have confirmed that women are more inclined to be submissives and men more inclined to be dominants, there are many exceptions to this.

Understand that not all BDSM "plays" end up in sex; some don't even involve touching each other. It is all about reaching orgasmic pleasures through taking control and surrendering (It depends on the role.). Most people in the BDSM scene do end up having intercourse, but it's definitely not required. Everything depends on your agreement with your partner or playmate on what you think is acceptable and interesting. Most of all, it is about consent.

Although this entire book centers on the role of the submissive, some light is shed on the other role—that of the dominant—for clarification purposes only.

The Roles

The dominant, or the Top, is often the one who takes control of the play. They are the one who sets up the play and "does things" and orders the submissive around. The Dominant should be someone you trust and someone who can take control of the situation. The person taking on the role must be sure of themselves and also knowledgeable on what is acceptable to the submissive.

Now to the meat of the matter, *the submissive*—the submissive is often seen as the one who aims to please their dominant, the one who likes being ordered around and do what they are told. There are people who naturally take to being submissive partners or have submissive traits that they carry around with them through everyday life.

The willingness of the submissive to do as they are told stems from an innate desire to please and serve another, typically someone they value or look up to. They are what are called True Submissives within the BDSM community. This means their submissive behavior is hard-wired into their brains. That is just how they are. To the True Submissive, being the servant, slave, or pet is not a role they play; it is who they are and there are no others roles they can fulfill.

There are also those in the community called Switches. Switches are people who can switch between being dominant and submissive in between plays and who play each role effectively. This also means that they are neither true dominants nor true submissives, but take on roles in the play.

How do you know if you are the Submissive?

As it happens, if you are interested in BDSM, or perhaps your partner has shown interest, and you want to try and see if being the submissive will fit in with your personality, you have to take a look into your own psyche. There are a few guide questions that can help you gauge your own personality. You will need to be totally honest with yourself. Try to give answers that reflect your real preferences rather than answers that you think you could fall into eventually.

Does serving another person, particularly someone you care for and love, make you happy?

Serving another can mean a lot of different things. A waiter serves, but so does a soldier. In the BDSM spectrum, serving pertains to doing something for the pleasure or benefit of another, the Dom. If you find yourself inclined to being helpful and of service to those around you, and that gives you genuine enjoyment in itself, then you just might be a Sub.

Are you inclined to sacrificing your own time and comfort for the benefit of others without thinking twice about it?

Do you go out of your way and spend time and effort just to be able to do something for someone else's benefit? Would you give up your free weekend just so a friend of yours can go on a vacation with her husband while you babysit their kids? If it makes you happy to sacrifice yourself for the sake of other people's happiness, then you could be a submissive.

Are you generally indecisive and do you find yourself easily swayed by others in making important decisions?

Try to look back in your life and see how many times you've had to make important decisions on your own and how many times you felt like you needed others to advise or help you. How did making decisions alone make you feel? Did making decisions on your own make you feel anxious and stressed, or was it easy for you? If you find it difficult making important decisions alone, then you might be a submissive.

Other quick questions to ask yourself:

When in a chaotic and confusing place, do you instinctively look for someone who can instruct you on your course of action?

Would you avoid confrontation rather than stand up for your ideas and beliefs?

Does having a partner who takes control in the bedroom excite you?

The questions above can only be used as guides in finding out if you have traits that may be submissive, but finding out if you are a true submissive is a difficult and complicated thing. Being submissive means complete surrender of control over what is happening. You are handing over the reins to a Dom, hopefully someone you love and trust who will do everything in their power to satisfy you as well. You have to be happy to give up control and follow orders. Even if you say yes to all the questions above and yet you are still uncomfortable with complete surrender of control, then you might not be submissive after all.

Chapter 2: How to Get Started as the Submissive

There are people who believe that it is the Dominant who is solely responsible for whatever pleasures can be gained from BDSM, but they couldn't be more wrong.

Although it is the Dominant who controls the play, the play will not be effective if you have a halfhearted Sub or one who tries to take control from the bottom (also called Top to Bottom). The submissive has to be responsible for themselves in every aspect and also give themselves up to the parameters of the play.

You, as the submissive, are just as responsible as the dominant in making sure you reach the heights of pleasure in your play. If this is your first time, it would be best if you have a dominant who has had some experience and is someone you trust.

Set the Scene

What is a scene? The scene for your BDSM play is like a story, a play, or, most commonly, a fantasy that you want to act out. Setting the scene will help guide you in reaching your goals and desires within your play. It is important to emphasize safe, sane, and consensual when setting up your play; this means the play itself has to be agreed upon and limits and parameters have to be set before you start.

The first thing to do when setting up a scene is to agree on why you are doing the scene in the first place. What do you want out of the play? Do you want to try new things and explore boundaries, or do you want some light fun and excitement? This has to be agreed upon before you start.

Once you know the parameters you will be confined (or not be confined) in, it is important to set up the story or fantasy as well as the progression of your scene. You have the option of simply talking it out or writing it down as you would a script for a movie. You and your dominant should have a clear agreement of what is going to happen, but if you, as the submissive, want to have a few surprises thrown at you, make sure your dominant is clearly aware of what is within the bounds of being acceptable.

Costume is also important in setting up a scene. It is best to wear clothes that reflect the setting of your fantasy as well as the roles each of you decide to play. The more accurate the costume, the easier it is to get into character.

Another important aspect of setting the scene is the location. In order to truly immerse yourself in your role play, it is important that you have a set location already. Most would have a private "dungeon" of sorts to do this or even a fetish club, but there are scenes that start out in public and end in private. Whatever you choose, make sure it is a safe environment for yourself and for your partner.

Have a Plan

As mentioned above, a scene is like a story or play. It follows that it should have a beginning, a middle, and an end, and it follows that you should have a plan in how your scene will unfold. This is where the Dom's experience is important. If you are both new at this, then you should definitely have a clear step-by-step outline of how the scene will unfold. More experienced Dominants can play it by ear, but even then, they should have a rough draft of what should unfold and when so that the play itself runs smoothly.

Make sure you have a clear understanding of what should transpire, whether there will be spanking, bondage, flogging, or whatever else.

Communicate as the Submissive

Even though you are the submissive, do not think even for just one second that you are passive. You are an active participant in this pleasure, and you have actively chosen your role in it. You went into this play and acted in this scene so that your desires can be achieved as well; it just so happens that your desires and fantasies are catering to the wishes and whims of another.

It is important that you and your Dominant have clear communication on what you both want out of this experience. Parameters have to be set, and that includes safewords. Make sure your safeword is something out of the ordinary that you would not normally say within the scene so that it cannot be overlooked by the dominant. If you intend on using gags or if you are doing your scene in a particularly loud place, make sure you have a signal you can use to communicate.

The most important aspect of these plays is SSC: safe, sane and consensual. You, as the submissive, have to be comfortable in the situation and in what the Dominant wants you to do or wants to do to you.

Chapter 3: Tools and Toys for the Submissive

There are a lot of toys and tools you can use within your play that can be both exciting and fun. However, it needs to be stressed that you should have prior knowledge on what you want to do and to what extent. There are ways to use these tools and toys that can be light and fun, as well as ways that could test your limits and take the scene to extremes.

You and your dominant should have experience and training in how to use some of the more complex equipment, such as bondage, piercing, scarring gear, etc. You should also be familiar with the risks that go along with these tools and know how to care of yourself and each other afterwards. Make sure you keep your equipment and toys in good condition to avoid accidents and mishaps.

Bondage Gear

Bondage play is when the Dominant restricts the Submissive's mobility and movement. Commonly, bondage gear is used to restrain the arms and legs, but it can also be used to reduce movement of the neck, feet, hands, head, and torso, depending on what you and your partner have agreed upon. There are many different kinds of Bondage gear, but the more basic and simple ones will be described here.

Cuffs

These include hand cuffs, wrist cuffs, thumb cuffs, ankle cuffs, thigh cuffs, as well as shackles and zip-ties, all of which are used to restrain the extremities. These are often the go-to gear for those looking to experiment or those who are new to the BDSM scene.

Collars

Though they may seem to be purely aesthetic, the collar is a good bondage toy that can effectively immobilize the head and neck, even the torso, especially if attached to furnishings or other equipment. You can choose to have a customized collar and have D-rings attached so that immobilizing can be achieved easily and safely.

Things to remember: Make sure that the cuffs or collars aren't too tight or that you don't go through more discomfort than you were bargaining for in the first place. The risk of postural asphyxiation, or just plain asphyxiation, is real, which is why constant supervision is needed. Remember that wrists, ankles, and especially the neck can be very vulnerable so take every precaution and make sure that you are SAFE. Make sure you have the correct gear for whatever you plan to do, as the quality of cuffs can go from almost useless to the really good quality leather kind.

Lastly, make sure you and your dominant know what you are doing. Don't try any ambitious positions that you are not familiar with as doing so can lead to consequences for which you might not be prepared.

Impact gear

Impact gear pertains to the items used in BDSM that involve striking at the submissive's body, often to cause pain but not all the time. There are those who go into impact play not for the pain but for discipline, subjugation, for the sound it makes against the skin, or even for humiliation. Impact toys have different effects and purposes and the intensity can range from not painful at all to extremely painful.

Floggers

The flogger is probably the most widely known of all impact toys. It is a short-handled whip that has many strips of leather. It can also be called a scourge or a lash. These are mostly made of good quality leather, but there are a myriad of designs out there that use other materials.

Floggers don't usually cause much pain—that is, unless you want them to. Again, the intensity of your play depends on the agreed upon parameters of your scene.

Paddles

The paddle is another common impact toy, and most are designed in a rather straightforward manner. It is usually a short wooden plank or any other hard material with a wide end and a handle. Unlike the flogger, the paddle has quite a lot of safety concerns that come along with it.

There are those who, in the heat of the moment, can end up hitting the submissive with the edge of the paddle rather than the flat surface. Also, striking the paddle at an angle can make the impact far more painful and damaging than expected, as the impact is no longer distributed throughout the surface of the skin.

Things to remember: Make sure that you do not break the skin. Check the flogger's tails to see if there are any foreign objects that can cause bleeding or break the skin, and make sure your paddle has a smooth surface. Hit only the muscled and fatty areas of the body and, if you are beginners, make sure that you start at the lowest intensity and amp it up as you continue to acquire experience.

While what is listed above are just a few toys that may be brought into play, you need to know that the dominant is probably going to be the one that makes the decision in making toy purchases so that the submissive does not know about anything new that may come into play. This also assists in adding to the element of surprise for the submissive because they never know what is going to happen during a session.

Sometimes there may be a mutual agreement in what is bought, especially if you are trying something new. It all depends on the relationship dynamic and who buys the toys.

Some of the most basic tools (some were discussed above) are:

-   Things for hitting such as paddles
-   Collars
-   Blindfolds
-   Leashes
-   Vibrators
-   Cuffs
-   Anal plug
-   Rope

But, there are other things that may be bought depending on the fetishes that you both enjoy.

-   Latex
-   Steel bondage items
-   Gas mask

- Straight jacket
- Arm binders
- Hoods
- Shock toys
- And more.

The most important part is that you have fun when you are purchasing and using toys. If you do not think that you are going to enjoy what is bought for you, make sure that you tell your dominant so that he can ensure that he does not use that type of toy on you and make you feel uncomfortable during a scene.

Chapter 4: Being a Good Submissive

Despite the fact that you may be a true submissive, there are still certain traits that you need to develop to be a great submissive and for you to find yourself in a healthy D/s relationship. The D/s relationship is already about submitting control to the Dom, and for a person with a True Submissive personality, abuse and bad relationships can be ever-present problems. If you find that you are a true submissive, there has to be a good balance of being submissive and getting what you want *and only what you want.*

The following chapter will be about certain traits that are needed in order to be a good, active sub in your relationship or play. As a sub, you have to realize what the essence of your role is as well as what you should bring to the table when you enter into a BDSM relationship.

Have a Healthy BDSM Relationship

There are certain things that are always needed in relationships, but there are certain particulars when it comes to a BDSM relationship, whether it's a real-life relationship that involves BDSM or a purely sexual BDSM arrangement. No matter what kind, it still requires some effort from both parties.

You and your Dom will need to be able to communicate with each other effectively. For your Dom to be able to do the right things and make the right decisions, you have to get your views and opinions across in a clear way and they have to be sensitive enough to truly understand what you mean. You both have to be willing to exert effort in making the relationship work and continuing to improve your immersion and play. Remember that a D/s, SM relationship is essentially the same as a vanilla (or "normal") relationship—it is the responses to conflict, the clearly defined lines on the roles each person plays, as well as the emphasis on respect and consent that make the BDSM relationship different.

To be a good Submissive...

- *You should have a clear desire to submit.* Honestly answering the questions listed in Chapter 1 is a good way of finding out if you have submissive traits. Being submissive does not mean that you like being a doormat, though, and being such can only lead to abusive relationships that cause pain and suffering. Being a good submissive means that you are your own person and you can still stand up for yourself; you just happen to want to relinquish control in the bedroom or (for some) even outside, but even then, only to a person (or persons) whom you choose, with the parameters of submission agreed upon between you as equals.

- *You need to be emotionally stable and to objectively assess yourself in the relationship.* As mentioned before, the traits of a true submissive, especially if they are not aware of such traits themselves, can be easy pickings for people who have less than honorable intentions and can make the submissive fall into abusive and manipulative relationships. This is why it is truly important to have emotional stability before seeking out a BDSM or, specifically, a D/s relationship. Don't go into the BDSM scene looking to be rescued by a princely Dom or for a Dom to find salvation through you. Try to take the time and review your past relationships and remember to be honest with yourself when trying to assess what went wrong. Being unable to be honest with yourself only means that it will be even harder for you to be in a relationship that requires honesty and communication, as all BDSM relationships do.

- *You should not be afraid to ask for whatever you might want or need from your Dom.* Although you are giving your Dom control over you, you have to realize that they are not mind readers who automatically know what you want and what you're missing. This is why communication is so important within BDSM relationships. It is a great help to the Dom to know what you want and it can help them anticipate your wishes rather than you sulking whenever your Dom misses the mark. The lines of communication should always be open between you and your dom, and you should never hold back in saying what's on your mind or in asking for what you want.

- *Submission should be your continuous choice.* A submissive in a healthy BDSM relationship should have the right to choose what they are submitting to, and choose to submit every day, every hour, even every minute as it happens. Your reactions and obedience are always your choice and you should not feel like you are being forced to do anything, although it may seem this way in the play. If you often feel like you are being forced to do things you are not comfortable with and don't necessarily consent to, then it may be time to reevaluate the rules and parameters of your relationship with your Dom, and even end it if you think it is necessary. All relationships, even BDSM, are give and take, and what is acceptable and unacceptable should be clearly defined between you and your Dom.

Although the character traits mentioned above are generally what one needs in order to be a good submissive, realize that all relationships, just as all people, have unique traits. The only thing to really watch out for is that everything in your play and your relationship is safe, sane, and consensual.

Chapter 5: The Different Types of Submissive Roles within BDSM

BDSM and role play have very defined sets of rules and roles for everyone who participates in them. The dominant has many different roles he can take on, such as Master, white knight, and demi-god, and all have different ways of being explored and handled. This is the same with Submissives. There are different types of roles that can be played by a submissive within a BDSM relationship or play.

Every type of submission has different parameters and it would be a good idea to have some basic knowledge of what the common ones are and what is often expected from such plays. Again, remember to have clearly defined rules and agreements on what is acceptable between yourself and your Dom.

The Brat

The submissive character of the Brat is the least understood character in the submissive's repertoire. The Brat is often characterized as being a generally obedient submissive but uses disobedience, teasing, and bad behavior part of the D/s play as a way to get punishment, attention, or discipline from the Dom. The brat can only be a good part of the D/s dynamic if it is an approved part of the play and not just a sub being difficult.

Being a brat in a BDSM relationship where it is not approved of by the Dom, or it is something a Dom is not capable of handling, is not indicative of a true submissive. It is what is often called "Top from Bottom," or a submissive trying to take control through manipulation. This is not fair and is actually frowned upon within the community. However, if the Brat behavior has become an integral part of the D/s, BDSM dynamic, then it is a dynamic that has to be reevaluated a lot. How much disobedience and to what extent it will be tolerated within the relationship is something the Dom and the Sub have to agree on.

The Slave

One of the more commonly known types of D/s is the Master/Slave dynamic. As a slave, the sub gives up control of every aspect of their life. They cannot own property or make any sort of decision for themselves. Submissives who take on Slave roles often give up control indefinitely, 24 hours a day, 7 days a week, to their chosen Dom or Master. Being a slave is a totally immersive experience and truly is a lifestyle choice, although there are those who do test out the waters. Those in master/slave relationships may function normally outside the home and return home to their BDSM play right away.

It is in this relationship that participants can truly explore their dark desires in many aspects, such as pain, humiliation, and sexual pleasure. It is important to remember, however, that a slave chooses to be a slave and should never be forced to do anything they do not want. This is why safewords and signals have to be clear and parameters have to be defined.

The Pet

The Pet submissive dynamic is a relatively easy and simple dynamic that is a good way for a novice submissive to get started in the BDSM scene. The pet often takes on the role of a beloved animal companion. This is a less immersive play and a pet submissive can slip in and out of character when needed. Also, pet play allows for some disobedience and mischief from the pet and is a good way to start out when you are new to BDSM. The Dom often takes on the role of owner, trainer, caretaker, etc., while the Subs generally fall into three main characters: the puppy, the kitten, and the ponies.

Kitten play means that the submissive displays certain feline characteristics and even a hint of independence; Puppy play centers around playfulness, mischief, collars, and leashes; whilst Pony play can involve riding (or at least simulated riding) and wearing bright plumage and carts. Although it can happen, most pet play has no sexual implications. Pleasure is derived from the attention and control your Dom gives you.

The longer you stay immersed in a submissive character, the stronger your will should be. You have to be sure of who you are and what is acceptable to you. It can be easy to lose yourself in the role play and subjugation, but remember that it is still your choice and your body.

Chapter 6: What to Watch Out For

So it happens that you are a submissive who has found her Dom and you have a certain dynamic going. That is all well and good, but it must be said that the BDSM relationship tends to be much more complex than the usual vanilla relationship. There are power plays and defined roles that have to be considered and taken into account.

Understand that these may or may not become problems for you in your particular situation, but it is probable that they become such. This chapter will focus on possible pitfalls and speed bumps you may encounter in your BDSM, D/s relationship.

Problems Trusting

When you are in a dynamic that asks for your complete surrender of control, it is important that you have complete and utter trust of your dom and vice-versa. Trust is never easy to give out and achieve, however, and having trust issues in your D/s relationship can hurt you and destroy the dynamic you've built. Thus, make sure that your Dom is someone worthy of your trust as well. And if he has proven or if you've seen signs that make you doubt them, then it may be time to get out of the relationship. It is also imperative that you go into the business of trusting. You have to know what you are both looking for in the relationship and what control and submission you are both willing to let go and give out.

Undefined Concepts and Rules

Although this has been heavily emphasized in this book, there are still many BDSM couples who fall into plays and scenes that take them by surprise or make them realize that they have fallen into a relationship to which they did not give their full consent. There are even times when the submissive starts taking control, leaving the Dom shaking their head. All this can stem from a lack of communication and defined parameters that are so important in all BDSM relationships.

The concept and the roles to be played have to be clear with both parties so that you can have a truly immersive play that satisfies the needs and wants of both.

Agendas

Whether in a D/s relationship or a vanilla relationship, there will always be instances when one person has a hidden agenda that can often lead to pain and suffering for one or both in the relationship. A hidden agenda does not necessarily mean making a clear plan and scheming against a partner. Sometimes, the person with these agendas is not even aware of what they are doing and how it affects the relationship.

There are Doms who end up abusing and manipulating their Subs without realizing it and Subs who take control and manipulate their Doms without really knowing what they are doing. The best way to avoid getting hurt in situations like these is to know yourself completely, know your wants and desires, know your limits, and know what you are willing to do. If you have a clear definition of who you are and what you want, then there is little chance that others can manipulate you and make you do things you'd regret.

Whatever problems you may encounter, always remember that even if you are giving up control as the submissive, it is always your CHOICE to submit. Your submission is a gift you are giving your Dom because you trust, respect, and/or love them. Never belittle the strength you have in you as a submissive.

Chapter 7: Getting into A Submissive Mind Frame through Training

Not everyone is going to agree while how submissives are trained. But, it is between the submissive and her dominant and how they are going to go about getting the proper training for the submissive so that she or he is able to do what is necessary to make the dominant happy.

Human psychology

There is part of the human psychology that is being shaped when you are working to train a submissive. The people that you are around every day are being trained even if we do not do it on purpose so that decisions are made in such a way that the result that is delivered is what is wanted. This is what submissive training is going to do because as a dominant, they are going to spend a lot of time with their submissive.

When you go through submissive training, you are going to be having your behavior changed to match what behaviors that the dominant wants and get rid of or discourage those that they do not want. With patience, the way that a person acts can be completely changed so that they are someone that your dominant wants to be around twenty four seven. However, it is extremely important to make sure that both parties consent to what is happening! This is extremely important when it comes to submissive training because this is the ultimate power exchange due to the fact that a dominant is getting into the submissive's mind and molding it to how they want it.

Training now days is not as bad as it used to be. In the old days submissives were beaten to get the behavior out of them that they do not want. Now, it is done more subtly such as a sigh or a facial expression. This does not just happen in a dominant submissive relationship, it also happens in vanilla relationships.

Kink therapy

For dominants and submissives alike, the power exchange can be extremely therapeutic. For a submissive, it is because they are not having to worry about their everyday worries. They are able to go to a different place and be someone that they are not in their everyday life.

Three aims for a submissive

As a submissive there are three goals that you are going to want to get out of their training in being a good submissive.

1. Behavior development: as a submissive you are going to want to get rid of any behavior that your dominant does not like. The faster that you get this done, the better your relationship is going to be. It will be hard to change behaviors that you have done for most of your life, but it can be done.

    When going through the act of training, you need to make sure that you are being trained by someone who is qualified in the skills that your dominant is wanting. There are schools that are going to be able to train a submissive that are going to teach a submissive all of the techniques that are desired by a dominant. Some of these qualities are:

    - Interpersonal skills

    - Management of a household

- Event coordination

- Personal attendance

- Organization and communication for business

- Sexual service

Dominant's personal preferences

You are going to want to be trained to your dominant's personal needs and preferences. Not every dominant is the same just as not every submissive is the same. Instead of just sending them to a school to learn the most basic of submissive skills, a dominant may take it a step further and send their submissive to a yoga class in order to improve flexibility and more.

Some other things that a dominant may want their submissive to know are:

- food preparation

- specific rules for specific situations and the consequences for breaking those rules

- schedules for work and personal life

- fetishes that are preferred by the dominant

- and how to do the proper massage without harming their dominant

Personal goals

Even as a submissive you do not ever want to quit growing. You are going to want to set goals that are going to help you grow and become a better person as well as a submissive. For example, if you are not happy with how you look, then you can enforce a diet to make sure that you can get to how you want to look and your dominant should assist with that. Or, talk to your dominant about making space and time for you to do a hobby that keeps you centered so that you do not act out.

A submissive's role

Every person has a different desire to be a submissive. There are four different reasons as to why a person may become a submissive.

- Selflessness: they want to please someone else and do not necessarily want anything in return.

- Active service: a submissive that participates in active service means that they are doing things for others such as cooking or managing a schedule if that is what is asked of them.

- Independence: being a submissive does offer a bit of independence because you are not necessarily having to deal with everything on your own. There is someone there that is going to assist you in making sure that things are taken care of. To the degree that they go in assisting is going to be between the dominant and the submissive.

- Passive service: if something brings pleasure to someone else and it involves them, then the submissive will do it. So, if flogging the submissive brings pleasure to her dominant, then she will allow for it to happen.

Before you can figure out what kind of submissive you are, you are going to need to make sure that you are compatible in a dominant submissive relationship and that your relationship is going to be a strong and healthy relationship that goes in a positive direction. It will also depend on the amount of training that you are going to require to make sure that you are doing what your dominant is desiring.

Conditional training

The word conditioning means that something is brought to the state that the person desires so that it may be used. So, when you having conditional training done to you, you are being changed so that you are going to be meeting your dominant's desires.

Behavioral training is going to be when your behavior is changed inside of a particular environment and you are rewarded whenever you are doing the proper thing and punished when you are doing what the dominant does not desire.

When you are going through conditional training, you may be given stimulus that is going to either tell you that you are doing the proper thing or that you are doing what the dominant does not like and they want you to change your behavior. Your response that you get may become part of your everyday life, as long as it is inside of a stable environment.

Classic conditioning

When talking about classic conditioning, most people think of Pavlov's dog. Whenever Pavlov rang a bell, the dog knew that it was time to eat, thus each time that the dog heard the bell, he began to salivate and know that he was going to get food.

Now translating that to being a submissive, if your dominant taps his fingers against something when he is annoyed by what you are doing, you are going to know that you are doing something wrong and depending on your dominant, you may or may not know that you are going to get punished. So, each time that you hear your dominant tapping his fingers, you are going to know that he is annoyed.

However, when you take it to a more fun level, you may be conditioned to know that whenever you see your favorite toy, you are going to be tied down to the bed and played with. But, this can be a bad thing because if you just happen to catch a glimpse at that toy and your dominant did not set it out, you are going to be expecting what always comes with that toy and yet it is not going to happen.

Operant conditioning

This conditioning comes with rewards and punishments. When something is done that the dominant likes, then you are going to be rewarded, but if you do something that they do not like, you will be punished.

Some things that you do unintentionally may fall into this category such as the way that you speak to our dominant or your body language, you are going to want to talk to your dominant about these because you are not going to want to be punished for things that you cannot necessarily control.

Positive reinforcement

Positive reinforcement is given, it is something that the submissive is obviously going to enjoy, such as having an orgasm or getting their favorite treat. However, these reinforcements are only going to be given because they did something that they know they are supposed to do such as doing the dishes every night after dinner.

Negative reinforcement

The stimulus that is desire will be taken away. This does not mean that the submissive will always be punished because they made a bad decision, it simply means that the dominant is taking away a bad feeling as a reward for doing something good. So, for example, perhaps the submissive has to wear an anal plug for the entire day until they return home. An anal plug is uncomfortable thus making it something that is not necessarily good, but not bad either.

Punishment

Punishment should only come whenever a behavior needs to be discourage. The dominant to the submissive should never be using punishment as way to scare their submissive, if this is happening, then the submissive is not in a good relationship.

Positive punishment

A stimulus will be given to the submissive that is going to discourage them from repeating a particular behavior. So, pulling on a submissive's nipples because they said something that was not for them to say. P.S. this is only going to work if the pulling is not a turn on for the submissive.

Negative punishment

The positive stimulus is going to be taken away for the undesired behavior being carried out. A good example for this is that the submissive favorite sexual toy is taken away from them for a determined amount of time that the dominant sets forth. Essentially it is like being grounded as a teenager!

Chapter 8: Communication is Key!!!

The proper dom is going to make sure that their submissive feels comfortable talking to them because they are not mind readers. However, communication can be difficult for a submissive, and this is going to come even more if they are wanting to talk about something that is not necessarily going to be taken properly by the dominant.

But, even if your dominant does not want to hear what the submissive has to say, the submissive needs to feel comfortable talking about it because this is going to ensure that both parties are being kept safe.

Say it!

- It should not matter what you have to ask for, you need to be able to know that you are going to be able to say it without breaking your dominant submissive relationship. The dominant may hold the power in the relationship, but you would be surprised that even if you ask for it, you are going to get it as long as it is not going to harm you or the dominant. You may not get what you want on your terms, but in those cases, you are going to get it on theirs.

- It should be all about you! You do not want to tell your dom how to go about making their job but they can go about telling you how to do yours. Even so, you need to make sure that you can express how you feel about things that may make you feel inadequate, what you need, your feelings, or anything else that needs to be expressed. This is a good way to discover where your hard limits are.

- Do not lie. If you are not explicit about what is bothering you, then how is it ever going to change? Despite the fact that being brutally honest is hard for everyone, it has to be done because it will help keep you protected in the end.

Trust your instincts

- Be positive. Do not go into a conversation with your dom believing that things are not going to change. Also, do not go into it without any solutions to the problems that may be occurring. It is not up to your dom to figure out how to fix everything. This relationship is a team effort and your dom will be impressed that you had something to offer up to fix the problem.

- Be attentive. You should not ever let your shields down. You need to look for the signs that are going to tell you what you need to do in each situation. If your dominant is in pain because they just received bad news, telling a joke is not going to be the best in that time. Instead, you are going to want to comfort your dominant without overstepping your bounds.

- Trust. Your dominant should have your best interest at heart and make sure that they are not harming you. Some people are great about hiding their feelings and it is hard to believe that they are actually doing right by you. However, a dominant is not going to do something to harm you and thus you need to trust that they are not going to harm you intentionally. If you feel that you need to, talk to them about how they reacted to something that may have been out of line at the time.

But remember, your dominant needs a safe place too, so do not use them as a human journal unless you are willing to do the same for them.

Chapter 9: Safe Words

We just talked about how communication is key as a submissive. A safe word is equally as important. In case you did not know, a safe word is a word or series of words that are going to be used a BDSM scene that tells the dominant that the submissive has had enough and that play is supposed to be stopped. A safe word is going to be agreed upon before the scene ever starts and the only people who know what the word means are the submissive and the dominant.

There are traditional things that a submissive can say such as no or stop but that does not mean that the submissive is wanting the dominant to stop what he is doing. Thus, a safe word is going to generally be a word that is not said during sex such as tree, red, cat, or even safe word.

If the submissive is not able to say their safe word, then they can give a signal that tells the dominant that they have had enough and that they need to stop the scene. This is also a way that a submissive can allow their dominant to know that they are okay when they have reached subspace (we will discuss subspace in the next chapter).

A safe word does not just tell a dominant that their submissive is done with the scene, but it also tells them that their dominant is okay during play. The colors are used during play to allow the submissive time to tell their dominant that they are good to go and want more, or that things need to slow down a little.

During role play, safe words are going to be used once the submissive has dropped out of character. For example, if they are done with the scene, then they may drop out of character and call their dominant by their first name. Unfortunately for the submissive, doing this may result in disciple because the submissive broke their character as well as used their dominant's first name without warning. So, a submissive must be careful in what they are doing.

Inside of the BDSM community, a safe word is a must because it is an added layer of protection for safe play and that way one does not push the other past the bounds of their relationship. Depending on the relationship, the submissive may just use their safe word or they may make their dominant to keep track of how they are during play and use their own discretion as to when the scene should be stopped. But, in situations like this, the submissive is consenting to give up their right to not use a safe word and possibly be pushed further than they are wanting to be pushed. If you are residing in the UK, consent has to be given away before the scene starts in order to stop the submissive from going after the dominant legally.

Some people who are strong advocates for having a safe word are not necessarily going to use a safe word themselves and this is because they have gone above an experienced level of play and taken it even further. But, do not confuse these people who are not going to use a safe word at all and are going to be participating in a total exchange of power. However, when this type of relationship is being built, a safe word may be used so that trust can be built between the two.

After a safe word, has been used, then the entire scene should be stopped and all toys and restraints removed immediately. It is considered dishonorable and even immoral should the safe word be ignored by the dominant. Depending on where you live, if you ignore someone's safe word, then you may be brought up on criminal charges because you then harmed someone without their consent. That does not include what punishment you are going to receive from the community once they have discovered what you did.

Forms of safe words

Safe words are going to be the way that the submissive has the power to stop the scene when she has had too much and needs to either take a break or has found a hard limit and cannot go any further. Safe words are not going to be said in traditional sex settings and they are going to be words that are not going to be said that may easy be construed as something that they are not.

Depending on the relationship, there may be different levels of safe words that are said through a scene to allow a dominant to know that the submissive is safe and still wanting more or things need to slow down. This is the dominant's way of not having to stop the scene completely and ruin the mood for both people.

Using a safe word and its effects

Despite what may submissive's think, using a safe word is not a sign of weakness, it is a way to ensure that you are being safe during play. While pushing yourself past your typical boundaries is not a problem, pushing yourself too far is not something that needs to happen or else you can become severely injured and damage your relationship with your dominant.

On the other hand, the use of a safe word may cause a dominant to feel as if they have failed and did not read their partner correctly or they have gone too far and did not realize it. This is one of the reasons that there are different levels of safe words because a submissive does not want to make their dominant to feel as if they have done something wrong.

Safe words are meant to be a word that says that there is no fault on either party that it was said. And discouraging the use of the safe words is not something that should be done because harm can be done to both partner's in their trust of each other.

In the event that a dominant thinks that their submissive cannot handle a scene or is not going to use their safe word, then they are to speak up because they do not want to harm their submissive. If a submissive is adamant about the scene, then they need to ensure that they are going to use their safe word so that they are not harming themselves nor their dominant.

The last thing that a submissive needs to know about safe words is that there is such a thing as consensual non-consent that is going to be when a safe word is no longer used and the body language is going to be read. This is going to most likely occur in the event that a punishment scene is being acted out.

For example, if the submissive is getting a predetermined number of lashes, then their body language is going to be read by their dominant to make sure that they do not push their submissive too far. If it happens, that the entire number of lashes are not met, then that is what is going to happen because being safe is more important than the scene that is being played out.

Chapter 10: Subspace and Subdrop

There are two different places that a submissive goes during play, the subspace and then what comes up, obviously has to come down so that is when a submissive sub drops.

Subspace

This is also known as head space and is when a submissive is overtaken by the combination of pain and pleasure.

Adrenaline, epinephrine, enkephalins, and endorphins are released whenever a body is placed into a fight or flight situation. However, a submissive will experience this when they experience an impaired sense of ability, out of body sensations, and their pain tolerance is tested.

Every submissive is going to have their own unique experiences when it comes to subspace. Some of the most common effects that a submissive experiences are:

- Impaired vision

- Loss of communication skills

- Hallucinogenic state of mind

- Limpness in limbs

- But the biggest thing that they will feel is a detachment from reality.

The biggest thing that a submissive needs to make sure her dominant keeps an eye out for is that he is not taking it too far whenever the submissive has reached the sub space due to the fact that since the submissive may not feel their limbs and cannot communicate, the submissive can end up being harmed.

There are also the other side of that where the submissive becomes addicted to the high and is wanting more physical stimulation so that they can stay in sub space longer. This is where a dominant is going to need to bring his or her submissive down because if he or she is not careful, then harm can be done and the submissive is not going to be able to tell reality from play.

Levels of subspace

- There is the ordinary level of head space

- The shift where the submissive begins to focus on the dominate and is more open to what they are told to do along with the dominant focusing on the submissive.

- "smart-assed masochist": this is where the submissive becomes disobedient and begins to challenge the dominant. A submissive may do this to test the dominant in order to see if they are going to actually do what it is that they say they will do if disobeyed.

- Blond space: the breathing is going to become deeper and the submissive may not be completely responsive to what is going on around them. This can come in the form of them forgetting orders, not speaking coherently, and even being overly giggly.

- Subspace: the submissive does not register all pain and the submissive may even lose consciousness.

- Flight or fight: the submissive loses all connection to reality.

Coming down

Whenever the body begins to stop the production of the chemicals that were mentioned earlier, then things are going to start coming back and it may appear as if the submissive is drunk or hung over. The sub drop can happen for a submissive inside of a few hours all the way up to a few weeks. It is imperative that the dominant take care of the submissive in order to make sure that there are no harmful feelings that are felt.

Dominants also experience a thing that is like subspace but it is known as dom space and they also experience coming down much like a submissive does.

Chapter 11: After care

Even though a dominant is going to usually be the one who administers the after care, it is best that the submissive knows what after care needs to be there and that she can do after care on the dominant as well.

After care comes in the techniques of pampering his submissive so that they understand they are cared for and that they are not along in a vulnerable state. Before a scene is played out, there has to be talk of after care so that the proper after care is given to each person. The amount of after care is going to depend on the scene that was played out and the dynamic of the relationship.

Benefits of after care

After care is meant to make the submissive feel safe and secured but also as a way to bond with their dominant. This is going to assist in eliminating the drop that many submissives feel when they are coming out of sub space.

Standard after care

No one can tell you that after care is being administered incorrectly because after care is going to based on the couples. However, here are some things that you can go through with your dominant to ensure that after care is being taken care of.

- Negotiate: talk about how after care is going to be administered so that there is no guessing by either party.

- Carry out play

- Once the scene ends, the dominant should switch to a nurturing state and take care of the bottom. The bottom needs to make sure that they are aware of what is going on.

- The dominant is going to take care of any wounds that may have happened during play and remove any restraints. As a blind fold is removed, it should be done slowly so that there is no shock to the bright lights of the world around them.

- Bottoms need to move to a warm and comfortable location with the assistance of the dominant.

- The dominant needs to make sure that the submissive is taken care of and that blankets are in reach so that when the temperature drops the submissive has something warm.

- Water should be nearby and it should not be out of something that is going to be difficult for the submissive to drink out of because they may not be completely able to move their limbs. Water should not be forced on the submissive.

- Positive reinforcement should make the submissive feel peace

- Touch for the submissive in ways that were not done in the scene play. The touch should be considered intimate and hypersensitive rather than torturous.

- Chocolate should be kept near by because it helps to release Oxytocin and stabalize the blood sugar.

- After care should continue up until the submissive is able to take care of themselves once again and they are in a good space in their head. The submissive should never be left alone to fend for themselves just in case they fall and harm themselves.

- Both the dominant and the submissive should be in a positive frame of mind before the part ways.

After care for the dominant

After care does not just go to the submissive. There is some level of after care that the dominant needs to recieve in order to make sure that they are okay about what happened in the scene as well. Mostly a dominant is going to take care of the submissive. A dominant should never play so hard that they are unable to take care of their submissive. However, should this happen, there should be a third party that is there to take care of both parties in the after care.

The same after care is going to be administered to a top as it is to a bottom however where a bottom is gonig to have specific needs based on what happens in the scene, a dominant is not going to necessarly have those needs.

Babysitters

There are going to be times that a dominant is not able to take care of their submissive all through the after care. In this case, there needs to be a third party that both parties have agreed upon that is going to take care of the submissive after play. But, the dominant needs to spend at least fifteen minutes with his submissive to ensure that he or she is not feeling abandoned right away. Doing this will cause the submissive to feel as though the dominant does not care and it will damange the relationship between both parties.

After after care

Once both the dominant and the submissive have been taken care of, after care does not does not just stop hours after the scene has ended. There are times that it can take up to several days.

To make sure that both parties are being given the proper support, they are going to reach out and communicate with each other about any feelings that they are feeling towards what happened.

If at any point in time that there are negative mood swings, they should be reported so that the proper support can be given.

Criticisms

Not everyone is going to want the same amount of after care. Everyone has their own form of after care the important thing is to make sure that both people can agree on after care and that it is adminsiterd in a way that is benificial to both parties.

Chapter 12: Tips to Be a Good Submissive

Everyone needs help from time to time and that is okay. However, it is what you decide to do with the help that you recieve that is going to define how good you become at your trade.

Being a good submissive means that you are going to have to put yourself into a particular mindset that is going to allow you to not only accept disicpline but to disicpline yourself as well.

Here are some tips on how you can be a good submissive to your dominant and be one that he is proud of.

1. Pick a good dominant: you need to make sure that you are not just getting into a dominant submissive relationship with anyone. This is a good way to get yourself hurt. Instead you need to get to know your dominant and the things that he or she enjoys so that you know if that is what you are willing to get into. If what they like are going to be hard limits for you and they are not willing to bend on these limits, then this is not the dominant for you. Remember, submissive is a choice and no one can force you into it!

2. Know your limits! You need to make sure that you know where you are not willing to go. This does not just mean mentally but physically and spiritually as well. These limitations are going to be where you are not willing to go and if a dominant cannot respect these limits, they are not the one for you.

3. Submitting means that you are giving everything that you have. As a submissive you are not going to just give up until you have had enough. A true submissive gives up until the

point in time that it hurts and even then they continue to give. A submissive is going to allow their dominant to know every inch of them inside and out. Also, giving your all will allow for your dominant to know how to be the perfect dominant for you.

4. You are not going to be perfect! You are human and you need to remember that. You are gonig to make mistakes and your dominant understands that. However, it is the fact that you need to be able to learn from your mistakes when you make them. A dominant is going to help make sure you are not harming yourself overmaking mistakes thus making you feel secure and safe.

5. Be honest. Your dominant is not going to understand when something has gone wrong because they are not able to read your mind. You have to tell them when something is wrong so that they can either fix it or help you to find a solution for it.

6. Do not be jealous. You cannot be jealous when you are in a dominant submissive relationship because it can kill your relationship with your dominant. It is very possible that your dominant will have more than one submissive and you have to be able to get along with that other submissive for the sake of keeping your dominant. However, the dominant needs to know how to keep each submissive separate because they are different and beautiful in their own way. If there is a chance that you are going to end up being jealous of another submissive, you need to discuss this with your dominant before you commit yourself to that relationship.

7. Obey your dominant. Even if you are a submissive that is going to lean towards disobeying, you need to try and always obey your dominant so that they know that you are willing to do whatever it is that they need you to do. The more that you obey, the more that you are going to be rewarded as well!

8. Your realtionship is not just about sex. What a dominant submissive relationship boils down to is control. There are some relationships that do not involve sex at all, instead they focus service between the two people. You need to make sure that you understand what it is that the dominant is expecting out of your relationship before you agree to commit to it.

9. Respect is a big thing in the world whether it be BDSM or not. However, a dominant is not going to tolerate disrescpect and you are bound to be punished if you do not show them respect!

10. While being a submissive is a choice, so is when you decide to be the submissive. You do not have to be a submissive all the time and just because you are a submissive does not mean that you need to be a doormat to those around you. You should only decide to be a submissive that you set forth with the dominant that you are working with.

11. There is no real true submissive. While it is often that said that a true submissive will do this or that, the biggest thing that you need to pay attention to is making sure that you are being safe and healthy in your relationship with your dominant.

12. You cannot allow your dominant to be the one to take full responsibility for your safety. You are the only one who

knows for sure when you are being harmed and if you feel like you are being harmed, then you need to speak up! Remember that you are an adult and you are putting yourself in this situation.

13. As discussed in a previous chapter, there are all kinds of submissives and it is your choice to pick which kind you are. If you do not identify with just one, then maybe you feel as if there are a couple that define who you are. That is not a problem just ensure that your domainant can handle the type of submissive that you feel like you are. You do not want a dominant that wants a toy when you are feeling like a baby girl. You need to find the dominant that fits you to a "T".

14. Support your dom, especially if you want them to be more involved in your daily life. Just like being a submissive, being a dominant can be scary and you need to support them just as they support you. So, offer your services when they are appropriate and make sure that you remember you are part of a team.

Conclusion

I hope this book was able to help you have a clear idea of what being a submissive really is and what it entails. You should now have a better understanding of what being a Sub in the BDSM, D/s world is really like and how safe and comfortable it should be for all parties i.e. dominants and submissives.

Hopefully, this book has been able to help you become more open and secure in whatever kind of kink or fetish you find yourself in as well as help you find a BDSM play or D/s relationship that is healthy and pleasurable for you and for the other party.

The next step is to live out your desires and dreams in a harmonious, safe, and comfortable environment with people whom you trust and respect, even love.

BDSM Playbook

The Secret Guide to Being the Dominant

Introduction

Thanks to 50 Shades of Grey, BDSM has gotten more attention than ever. Unfortunately, the novel doesn't really provide neither a comprehensive nor accurate look into the lifestyle.

If you are curious in finding out how BDSM works, and would like to be part of the community as a Dom personality, this book is for you! By the end of this book, you should have the firsthand knowledge and confidence to foray into the life of BDSM kink, and associate yourself with people who can teach you more!

Chapter 1: BDSM and the Community

BDSM stands for Bondage, Dominance, Submissive, and Masochism. It has gotten quite a reputation after the popularity of 50 Shades of Grey which gives a glimpse into the world of BDSM. However, the book and the movies don't really give an accurate presentation of how this lifestyle works. In this eBook, we'll offer you a rare look into how BDSM works, specifically on the side of the Dominant Role. Note that it's not all about lashings and being the "Boss" in the relationship. You'll find that as a Dom, you'll have to consider other factors in order to be accepted into the community.

Are You Sure You're Into BDSM?

Not just because you think it's hot to tie your partner up during sex does NOT mean you're into BDSM and take the role of a Dom. Try to make a list of what BDSM features you'd like to try out and introduce them to your partner. It's perfectly acceptable if you don't know exactly how BDSM will affect your overall sexual experience since for the most part, people have no idea how the lifestyle works. Generally speaking, BDSM does NOT have sex as its end result. The sex is simply incidental with the pain and discomfort being the primary goals.

If your goal, however, is sex but with a bit more action, then you're not really into BDSM. Chances are you still want sex, but what to make things more exciting. A little leather, a little bondage, and a little exercise in power are not a problem in sex, but it doesn't automatically translate to BDSM. That doesn't mean you shouldn't experiment, however, since you'll never really know unless you try.

Who Is a Dominant?

The Dominant is the one who takes control of the situation. More aptly put, this is the individual who decides what will happen inside the room. Traditionally, the dominant is the one who holds the whip, restraints, or inflicts pain on the submissive. Anything the Dom wants done is followed by the Sub under the cloak of no limitations. Of course, there are actually limitations, but having no limits as to what you can do is part of the fantasy. Typically, the Dom and Sub must talk about the situation before plunging into it beforehand.

Who Is a Submissive?

The Submissive or the Sub is the one who follows orders. They are the ones who are restrained, whipped, or who do whatever is requested by the Dom in the interest of role play. You'll understand later on that one of the hardest parts about BDSM is finding the perfect Sub who fits your personal preferences. For now however, it's important to first define the important qualities and roles of the Dom which will be discussed later.

BDSM Services

The BDSM community is popular enough that there are currently facilities catering to BDSM requirements. You have probably heard of facilities composed of several rooms where BDSM activities are held. These are special types of facilities that often offer an array of professional Submissive-types who will do your bidding.

Now the question is: how do you find these facilities in your community? We'll talk about that later in the Chapter. Of course, it's usually better if you find a sexual partner who is also happy to play the role of the Submissive.

The Community

The Community is fairly tight knit and despite the popularity of 50 Shades of Grey, the fact is that the BDSM lifestyle is still under much scrutiny. This is why it isn't surprising that the BDSM community stays low and is rarely advertised so blatantly. The internet is one of the best places to learn about the lifestyle but as for the real-world, you will need to be in contact with people in order to be part of it in the truest sense. BDSM functions much like a secret society wherein you have to meet the right people and prove your interest before being handed a passport or a map towards the center of the community.

One thing you should keep in mind is that being a closely held community, those who favor BDSM have made unofficial rules in the conduct of the Dom and the Sub for the control and protection of both. Many of these will be tackled later but for the most part, understand that there are certain regulations set forth under this lifestyle. The rules may vary from one BDSM facility to another, so it's up to you to learn what they allow and forbid.

Wait, So Is This Legal?

The short and simple answer is – YES. However, the intricacies of it can be quite complicated. Generally speaking, prostitution is illegal in the United States and prostitution is defined as the performance of a sexual act in exchange for money.

BDSM however, is not always about sex. In fact, within the regulated community, there is no sex involved and thus, no law violated. In fact, BDSM facilities go through the routine checks performed by the authorities to ensure that the building is up to code when it comes to fire hazards, earthquake, electrical wirings, and the like.

However, there are instances when BDSM has an element of sex added into it. If you are part of a BDSM Club made up of private people, then it's likely that the BDSM/Sex interplay is purely consensual with no exchange of money between the parties. If you and your partner also enjoy BDSM play within a committed relationship, then this should not be a problem.

Safety During Role Play

The first concern in BDSM is safety. Although inflicting pain and discomfort is inherent in bondage, the intention is to be able to do this without causing excessive injury to a person. Bearing in mind the different tools utilized in BDSM, it's not uncommon for Subs to go home with the beginning of a bruise on their skin – but as much as possible, the community wants to limit telltale effects to bruises on the skin. Blood and broken bones are best avoided and in all cases; instances of this will prompt the Sub to speak out the safe word.

Later on, this eBook will discuss how to perform the different facets of a BDSM Dom without going beyond the lines.

Learning the Language

BDSM is just not a community – it's a lifestyle, which accounts for the fact that they have their own language. Here's what you should know before diving into the community:

Adult toy chest/ toy bag

This is a person's collection of "toys". Usually it's the Dom who has this covered.

Alligator clamp

This is a kind of a nipple clamp that looks like an alligator jaw. Most alligator clamps have adjustable screws with rubber tips.

Animal Transformation Fantasy

This is when the sub assumes the role of different specie which can be a dog, a horse, or a cat. It can also be enhanced by *Animal Play* wherein the sub not only acts but also dresses up as the animal they're supposed to be.

Aftercare

This is an important part of every Dom-sub interaction after the play session wherein the two snap out of their roles and talk about the events that transpired and what they feel about it. This is important to help both the Dom and the sub to get back to normal levels.

Ageplay

This refers to daddy/daughter or mommy/baby situations. The focus here is not on incest but rather, on the nurturing aspect of the relationship. In some cases however, ageplay may also refer to relationships where there is a marked gap between the two participants. For example, a teacher-student role play is quite common for many.

Auction

Adding a bit of spice into the whole experience, an auction essentially involves the sub with Doms bidding for an individual they want to be their slave. Note that this is usually on a temporary basis.

Anal Torture

The act of inflicting pain on the anus.

Bad Pain

Bad pain is essentially the kind of pain that is not mutual or not consensual during the play. It must be kept in mind that BDSM involves pain – but such is consensual pain or within the bounds accepted by the sub or carry a purpose to the play. Anything beyond that is considered Bad Pain and should be avoided.

Ball gag

You insert this rubber ball into the submissive's mouth and hold it in place with a strap.

Ball torture

This may cause pain to a man's testicles, but you can adjust the pain level until the submissive gives in.

B &D, B/D, B/d

This stands for bondage and dominance.

BDSM

This is the acronym for **B**ondage and **D**iscipline, **D**ominance and **S**ubmission, **S**adism and **M**asochism.

Black Sheet Party

An orgy for people practicing BDSM.

Body art or modification

You alter a part of the body, for example, by drawing tattoos or branding a person. You could also pierce the skin, stretch, or inflict scars.

Bondage

Involves physical restraint of the sub, typically involving handcuffs or a tie and in some instances, it may be limited to just a certain body part, such as in Breast Bondage. This also refers to making the person helpless and partially immobilized. You do this by tying the arms and legs of your partner and making him/her submit to all the things you desire in bed.

Bottom

The sub (as opposed to the Top or the Dom).

Breath Control

Play wherein the Dominant takes control of the breathing of the sub.

Boot licking

You ask your partner to lick your (the Dom) boots as a sign of submission.

Branding

This is a permanent scar that Dominant puts on the skin of the submissive. You can do this by applying heated metal to the skin of your lover.

Brat

When a submissive tries to gain the Dom's attention by behaving like a spoiled child, he/she is called a brat.

Breast bondage

Men tie up or restrain the boobs. There are many sorts of contraptions for breast bondage.

Bullwhip

This is a long leather whip. It is also heavy.

Butt plug

You may use this for anal play, either for punishment or for entertainment. Either way, you place this toy in the anus of the submissive.

Cage

The submissive lover is in a cage, the smaller the better so that the submissive would not be able to move freely.

Charity

A form of orgasm denial. A person is prevented from achieving orgasm through the use of tools that stop the person from accessing their genitals. For women, this usually involves a chastity belt while for men, a cock cage.

Collared and Collaring

A collared sub is someone who is owned by a Dom in an intimate and loving relationship. Note though that this doesn't mean exclusive since the Dom can have several collared subs. Being collared puts the sub into a *pup* status as opposed to someone who is a *stray*. Collaring is the formal acceptance of a Dom, Master, or Trainer with respect to a sub.

Contract

It outlines the agreement between the Dominant and the submissive regarding their roles in the relationship. This isn't legally binding but sets the rules as to how each one is supposed to proceed in the relationship.

Caning

You use a cane, which is usually made of rattan, on a sub. Warning though: This could be extremely painful on the other person. This is worse than flogging.

Cat o' Nine Tails

This is a fancy term for a whip with nine tails. For added sensation, choose the one with beads or anything knotted on the whip.

CBT/ Cock and ball torture

This is the pain inflicted on the submissive's penis and/or testicles.

Chocolate

Any sexual activity that isn't vanilla is called 'chocolate'.

Clover nipple clamps

These are rubber-tipped or rubber-colored clamps that are connected by a chain. When you pull the chain, the clamps tighten and produce a wild sensation on the sub's nipples.

Coca-Cola submissive

This person obeys the rules of BDSM only when he or she feels she wants to obey them. Also acts like a brat.

Cock ring

You slip this ring around the base of the guy's penis so he could prolong his erection.

Collar

This is worn by the submissive to indicate that he/she belongs to the Dominant. It also means that the sub is the slave of the Top.

Corset

Popular in the old days, the corset gives the woman an hourglass figure. It also accentuates her breasts.

Crop

This is a type of whip used in horseback riding. It leaves a sting on the submissive.

Cupping

This increases the blood flow on a body part and adds sensation to the sub. To do this, place suction cups on the skin. You could also use your mouth to suck in the skin and 'brand' your slave.

D/s:

Dominance and submission.

Dom

Dominant or the one in charge. The one who holds the power in the sexual activity. He/She is the one who controls the play and tortures the submissive.

Dominatrix

The female version of a male dominant. Also called domme.

DM or Dungeon Monitor

This is the person who supervises the play in the dungeon to make sure that both parties stay within limits.

Dungeon

Room or area where the BDSM play happens. This is where the toys and equipment for BDSM are put up.

Edgeplay

These are forms of BDSM play that are on the edge or have the probability of causing harm, either physically or emotionally. It can be quite subjective since D/s has very varying perceptions of what is dangerous and what isn't. Often however, this includes fireplay, gunplay, bloodplay, and breathplay.

Erotic Spanking

Spanking the other party to stimulate sexual arousal.

Extreme restraints

This refers to a bondage device for extreme restraints and should not be used by beginners to BDSM.

Femdom

A female Dominant. This is another name for domme.

Fetish, fetishism

One's fetish is outside the "normal" things that you do in bed. This fetish gives you sexual gratification. For example, some dominants find a fetish in seeing blood in their submissive, so they cut a part of the skin.

Fisting

The Dom (male or female) inserts entire hand into the sub's anus or vagina.

Flagellation

You can stimulate your partner's genitals by whipping or flogging him/her.

Flogger

Often made of leather, the flogger delivers sting.

Freeplay

This is BDSM play but without a power exchange.

Good Pain

As opposed to Bad Pain, this is the kind of pain that is consented to by the other party and usually carries with it a purpose.

Golden Showers

Urination fetish whereby a person enjoys being urinated on or urinating onto another

Hard Limits

BDSM type of play that someone will absolutely NOT do

Hobble skirt

The hobble skirt gives the wearer less room for movement.

Kitten

Usually the term of endearment given to a submissive, also a role ascribed to the sub during animal fantasy.

Lash

This is a blow from an object with a flat surface, usually, like the whip, crop, or paddle.

Leather

Used for whipping and bondage. It is the common fetish in sex and BDSM because it is a very sexy material. It doesn't break too in extreme play.

Leg cuffs

These restrain the sub's ankles.

Limit (hard limits, soft limits)

This is the sub's final boundary. When he/she gives a soft limit, it means that something might change over time. If there is a hard limit, the sub will never permit a certain act.

M/s

This title stands for Master/ slave.

Master or Mistress

This is typically the word used by the sub when referring to the Dom during a scene. Hence, although the Dom is often referred to as "he" in this book, there are also female Doms.

Martinet

This refers to a small or French flogger.

Masochist

This is a person who finds pleasure in pain; the opposite of the sadist.

Munch

A BDSM meeting in a vanilla location or a location that is public and accessible to the public. This is often a social call with each other about past or future BDSM plays.

Nipple clamps

These are sex toys that you attach to the nipples, so they could stimulate the breasts of the wearer. The sub could experience both pleasure and pain.

Nipple torture

This means to make the sub's nipples painful.

Nipple weights

You add or suspend weights from nipple clamps for increased pleasure or pain on the sub.

OTK

This means over the knee, said when you want to spank a partner.

Paddle

This is a wooden or leather flat instrument that you use for spanking your sub.

Pet

This is another term of endearment for your sub.

Pony play

Common in animal fantasies, the sub takes the role of a pony (Which the Dom can ride, tether, or spank).

Power exchange

This is done when the sub willingly hands over control to the Dom for the play or for the rest of the relationship.

Prince Albert

This is a male piercing between the urethra and the penis.

Puppy play

The sub takes the role of a puppy.

Pussy torture

One causes pain to a female's vagina or clit.

ProDom or ProDomme

Professional Dominants charging money for their services.

PlayParty

A BDSM Party.

RPG/ Role play games

You take on various roles like doctor/nurse, teacher/student, and parent/child.

Red

Say this to stop all play.

Restraint

You limit the freedom and movement of your sub.

Ring gag

This is a ring attached to a strap to keep the sub's mouth open.

Rope

This is a usual type of equipment for bondage.

Rubber

This is another fetish material popular in BDSM, like leather.

_S&M, S/M_

These initials stand for sadism and masochism.

Sadist

A person who enjoys inflicting pain on their partners. They like to see their partners getting tortured because it gives them sexual gratification.

Sadomasochism

This is when a person who feels sexual gratification from sadism and masochism.

Safe, sane and consensual

This is the "slogan" or number one rule in BDSM.

Safeword

The word used by the sub if she wants to stop the scene. Red is the common safe word (like red light). Yellow, on the other hand, means the sub is about to say Red. If the Dom ignores the safe word, he/she is considered unsafe.

Saint Andrew's Cross

It is shaped like a cross and is used in BDSM. The sub is restrained against the Saint Andrew's Cross when the Dom uses this.

Scene

It is a session, a sexual activity between the Dom and the sub, which can be performed in private or in front of other people. It is also the time period for the BDSM play.

Slapper

This paddle produces a loud noise when it hits the skin.

Slave

This is another word for the sub.

Slave contract

When the Dom and the sub have a slave contract, it ensures that whatever act happens between them is consensual and legally unenforceable.

Switcher

This is the kind of person who can take both the Dom and sub role, depending on the scene.

Spanking bench

The spanking bench looks like a picnic table, but is used to restrain or limit the movement of the sub.

Spencer paddle

This is a paddle with holes to give more pain to the sub.

Spreader bar

This bar holds apart the body parts of a sub.

Stocks

The sub's hand and head go through holes while he/she is standing.

Strap-on

A dildo is attached to this belt.

sub/ subby/ subbie/ submissive

This is the person who gives in to the Dom during the power exchange. Also called a slave.

Subspace

This means the sub consents or allows himself to enter or act in a scene.

Suspension

You suspend the sub using harnesses, belts, ropes and chains. Beginners should not use this.

TPE/ Total power exchange

Total Power Exchange or a 24/7 relationship.

Top

The Dominant in a relationship or in a scene.

Topspace

The Dom's state of mind that he/she may participate in a scene.

Topping from the bottom

The sub tries to control the actions of the Dom.

Tweezer nipple clamps

Nipple clamps that look like tweezers.

Vanilla

Someone who is not into BDSM play, also sex that happens outside the BDSM, opposite of chocolate.

Violet wand

According to BDSM practitioners, the violet wand smells of "ozone". Actually, this is a device that sends electrical charges at contact so it could provide stimulation.

Wartenberg wheel

This is also a device that is used to apply sensation. It looks like a pizza cutter, only spiked.

Wax play

The Dom pours hot wax onto the sub's skin during play.

Whipping post

During play, the sub is tied to the whipping post.

Chapter 2: Role Play – The Submissive-Dominant Relationship

Later on, this eBook will discuss how to perform the different facets of a BDSM Dom without going beyond the lines. First however, it's important to talk about the Dom/sub Relationship.

Dom/sub Relationship

If you'll notice, the word Dom is always written with the first letter capitalized while the sub makes use of the small letter. This is in accordance with their roles wherein the Dom takes the Top spot and the sub is also the bottom.

Note that although the Dom is the one in charge, it is the sub that has the power to stop the scene. The Dom therefore needs excellent self-control that will allow him to stop when the sub asks for a reprieve.

Dom and Control

The Dom is the one in charge, but that doesn't make his job easy. In fact, the Dom has to have extreme control over his person and make sure that he doesn't go beyond the Hard Limits and the limits set by safety. He should always keep the welfare of the sub as his first concern while satisfying his personal pleasure. Remember that with BDSM, both the Dom and the sub get off on their particular roles; the trick is to find that balance wherein both of you get your pleasure without going beyond what is allowed.

Pre-Play

What you do before playing is every bit as important as what you do after. Typically however, a pre-play is done for paid-facilities wherein subs will want to find out the extent of your knowledge on BDSM, the kind of scene you want to play, the Hard Limits, and the Soft Limits they have for their person. Pre-Play is also where the Safeword is determined or any other symbol used for the safety of the sub.

Aftercare

Aftercare is often defined as the healing process after the BDSM scene. In fact, most people say that aftercare is part of the play scene and essentially helps the Dom and sub to go back to neutral level. This is because after the end of a scene, the Dom and sub are likely still buzzing over what happened. The Dom is still clinging to his Dominant personality while the sub is trying to recover from the emotional and physical hurdle she was exposed to. By going through aftercare, the Dom and sub manage to adjust their moods and emotional status and resume their original roles outside the dungeon.

Aftercare is incredibly important and is one of the factors that separate an excellent Dom from a bad one. More on how to practice Aftercare will be talked about later.

Safe, Sane, and Consensual

This is essentially the BDSM Mantra or the Golden Rule. It comes in many forms but the essence falls down into these three categories: Safe, Sane, and Consensual.

Safe in the sense that there should be safeguards put in place starting with the safeword, the use of BDSM-approved restraints, and even the presence of a monitor if need be. Sane relates to the purpose of the play. The pain or discomfort inflicted should be in relation to the scene or has a definite purpose. Inflicting pain without any viable reason attributable to the BDSM scene is a Bad Pain and should not be tolerated. Lastly, there's Consensual which means that the sub MUST CONSENT to the play or to the techniques being used in the play.

Chapter 3: Tools and Toys for the Dominant Role

BDSM leads to better sex

Great sex is when you can be free to be yourself with your lover -- no hang-ups, no pretenses. This is what you get with BDSM sex. Imagine how liberating it is to know that you're having sex with the *real* version of your partner.

Great sex requires variety and couples who practice BDSM are constantly expending time and effort in finding ways to make sex more exciting for each other. Trying one sexual adventure after the other enhances your curiosity and your confidence in bed.

Great sex is a result of great foreplay. Often in BDSM sex, there is constant touching involved. It's not the mindless, mechanical coupling that usually occurs during vanilla sex. In order for BDSM sex to work, it requires you to be aware, to be in the present, to be an active participant. And isn't that what a healthy relationship is all about?

BDSM leads to better communication in relationships

In order to have great sex, it's important that you don't just *do* it. You also need to be able to *talk* about it. Keeping all of your needs and fantasies to yourselves inevitably leads to dissatisfaction, frustration, and resentment towards each other. Couples who engage in BDSM are more communicative when it comes to expressing their sexual desires. In turn, they also become more open in expressing their deepest emotions.

In vanilla relationships, couples don't usually talk openly about sex. They don't confront their partner's shortcomings or wonder about their own until such a time when their relationship or marriage becomes threatened. BDSM couples, on the other hand, are naturally honest and direct with each other because they need transparency in order for the BDSM relationship to thrive. In fact, most BDSM couples tend to develop a secret language that only the two of them can understand. Each time you talk about rules and safe words or make a list of things that you want to do between the sheets, you are actively communicating and considering each other's needs.

BDSM increases intimacy between couples

When couples do something new together, this makes them vulnerable to each other. When you share an adventure with each other, the experience binds you. How can it not? You share a secret together. You've shared one euphoric moment after the next. Moreover, that feeling of bliss that you experience each time you try something new is automatically linked to your partner. Thus, when you think of each other, you end up feeling the exciting sensation all over.

This goes without saying but each time you let your lover bind you, or blindfold you, or flog you, it necessitates a high degree of trust which is essential in all relationships.

BDSM promotes fidelity

Contrary to what most people may believe, BDSM relationships do not often lead to lewd sexual behavior, multiple sexual partners, and infidelity. In fact, couples who take BDSM seriously end up investing a great deal of time, energy, trust, and emotion into the relationship that it would be less likely for them to do anything to sabotage their efforts. They are unlikely to risk all the trust and safety that they have painstakingly built. Furthermore, two of the major causes of infidelity are sexual incompatibility and stagnation. Both rarely apply in BDSM relationships.

BDSM aids in improving mental health

Studies reveal that BDSM friendly individuals are less fearful, more open-minded, more secure in relationships, and better at coping with rejection. According to research, BDSM has therapeutic effects to individuals who have experienced psychological trauma in the past. That's because it allows you to express your sexuality without fear or shame. BDSM sex requires you and your partner to be fully present: mind, body, and soul during the interaction and thus the therapeutic powers of BDSM can be likened to that of yoga or mindful meditation.

BDSM lessens psychological stress and anxiety

A scientific experiment revealed that while participating in BDSM activities, the subjects' stress levels have noticeably decreased. Both dominants and submissives reflected lower cortisol levels in their systems. That's because in BDSM sex, you let go of expectations and judgment to give way to physical intensity. While observing both sub and Dom subjects engage in giving and taking pain, scientists discovered decreased blood flow in the prefrontal and limbic pain regions in the brain. This yields a tranquilizing effect, thus lessening anxiety.

BDSM encourages self-advocacy

Who you are in bed is a reflection of who you are in real life. If you're frightened, anxious, or uptight between the sheets, that's who you are at home and at work. Whether or not it is manifested externally, it's who you are inside.

Participating in BDSM sex helps you become more honest and more upfront about your sexual needs. When you learn to confidently speak out in the bedroom by giving a command, that's when you stop being a person who just sits and wait for others to anticipate your needs. When you learn to speak a safe word during BDSM sex, that's when you stop becoming that person who's too afraid to interrupt someone mid-speech regardless of how uncomfortable you're feeling.

BDSM teaches responsibility

Whether you are a sub or a Dom, BDSM teaches you that you are responsible for the quality of your sexual experience. Being a dominant is not about taking advantage of your power to suit only your selfish desires just as being a submissive is not about shutting your brain off so you could let your partner do all the work. BDSM is all about establishing a give-and-take relationship.

Some people mistake the role of the submissive as a powerless position and thus, one that is free from any responsibility. On the contrary, there is a special kind of power that the submissive possesses over the dominant. It's the sub who decides how long he/she will continue to give away his/her control. The moment the sub uses the safe word, the Dom must stop. Once the submissive decides that he/she will no longer relinquish power, the Sub-Dom relationship is over.

Chapter 4: Safety and Techniques

Safety is the most important concern when it comes to BDSM play. As the Dom, you'll be the one to predict the scene and hold the control on how the play proceeds. The main protection of the sub would be the Safeword which may be uttered at any time to stop the play. This is usually done when Hard Limits are tackled. In the previous Chapter, we talked about the Dom-sub relationship and how to foster trust between the two. In this Chapter, we'll try to talk more about how to ensure safety during play.

Note that ensuring safety isn't all lodged onto the Dom. A good sub will be able to arrange herself in such a way that it minimizes any pain, injury or discomfort. As the Dom however, much is in your hands:

Safeword

The safeword can be anything and everything under the sun as long as it doesn't usually come up during the play session. For example 'no' and 'stop' are quite common in BDSM scenes, especially for those who have a fetish for begging and pleading play. The use of out-of-context words therefore become necessary to fully indicate that play time is over. For example, 'pineapple juice' and 'spongebob' are good safeword choices because they're unlikely to come up during the play.

Note though that safewords aren't always possible. What if you're engage in gag play and the sub can't talk? This is where specific actions or symbols come in. The sub may shake her head three times, nod her head three times, raise up three fingers, or push a button somewhere in the dungeon. The signal can be anything as long as the sub has easy access to it throughout the play.

Check In

A 'check in' is a technique to make sure that the sub still gives consent during the play. This is especially true if you happen to be in the middle of a flogging or perhaps starting a natural development to the play. You want to 'check in' with the sub to make sure that you're not going beyond what she allows. A check-in can be something as simple as asking the sub if she still remembers her safeword. This gives the implication that although she knows exactly what the safeword is, she has no desire to use it during the play. Of course, a 'check in' must be thoroughly explained with your sub before the play starts so that she doesn't accidentally blurt out the safeword when you ask.

Set Limits

After setting up a safeword for your sub to use, the next is to set up Soft and Hard Limits to be followed. Soft Limits are those that are subject to change. Perhaps the sub is curious about this type of play and will welcome it when she learns more about the procedure. Hard Limits however are absolutely no-go and will rarely be subjected to change. As a Dom, you should keep this in mind throughout the play.

Flogging, Spanking, and Planking

When it comes to floggers, cheap is definitely worse. The best flogs are those made from deerskin – they can be expensive, but they guarantee the least amount of damage. Cheap flogs can draw blood even when used with less force. Also note that there are danger areas when flogging. The upper back, thighs, and ass are usually the best places because they can be fleshy and are nowhere near vital organs. What you want to avoid is the face, the neck, the region near the kidneys, the stomach, knees, and elbows. These are generally Bad Pain areas in the community. Spanking and planking make use of the same rules and regulations as to where you should hit.

Using Gags

Gags are also a common element of BDSM play, but you have to be very careful when using them on your sub. Generally, a gag should NEVER encompass the nose because this makes it doubly hard for the sub to breathe. Make sure to use a gag that's soft on the skin to avoid abrasions.

Slapping

When hitting the facial area, slaps should be confined to the cheeks and nowhere else. Hitting the eyes, nose, and mouth can be dangerous for the sub.

Restraints

The first rule in restraints is that you should NEVER leave a restrained sub alone in the dungeon, even for a second! A restrained sub is incapable of movement and is exposed to numerous dangers without a Dom there to ensure that nothing bad happens. Remember that this is your play and even though you have a Dungeon Monitor, the Dom/sub is a very unique relationship so that you will be the one who has to remove the restraints. Note that restraints don't just mean ropes – they're also about handcuffs, silk scarves, or any kind of tying implement. It's best to purchase materials specially made for BDSM purposes to prevent abrasions on the skin of the sub.

Ideally, the restraints should be loose enough that they still allow blood flow through the body. A sub should always be on the lookout for tingly or numbing feelings along the limbs that are restrained. It is the role of the Dom to check in once in a while and make sure that there is no blood restriction occurring due to the bondage.

Collaring

Included in the area of restraints is the use of collars which isn't always advertised in BDSM. The truth is that collars can inhibit breathing which can lead to death. As much as possible, collars are discouraged in BDSM – however, if this is really your thing, then we strongly suggest the 'two finger' rule. This means that the collar has to be loose enough that you can insert two fingers in between the skin and collar without any problem. Anything tighter than that is dangerous.

Aftercare

During aftercare, the Dom manages to become more caring as a natural way of deviating from the Dominant mental status he goes into during the scene. The sub, on the other hand, experiences an emotional uplifting afterwards to help level the physical and mental pressure they went through. Here are some examples of how aftercare works:

- Taking a bath or shower together with the Dom administering to the sub in different ways like massaging shampoo or soap.

- Taking care of any cuts and bruises that the sub got through application of creams, band-aids, ice packs, and gels.

- Massaging any of the sore muscles.

- Food and water to rehydrate the body.

- Talking about what happened and allowing the sub to talk about the scene, in some cases involving cries, anger, or any method of self-expression.

- In some cases, the talk can be about what you liked during the scene and what you didn't like

- Cuddling with each other.

- Having sex at a gentler and more leisurely pace with your partner

- Talking about your feelings with each other and how much you love her

- Brushing her hair or applying lotion all over her body

Of course, those are just examples of aftercare. As a Dom, you should be mindful of the kind of aftercare your sub needs. The more stringent the scene played, the more extensive the aftercare should be. Remember that you're essentially the owner of your sub and although you can do what you want with her during a scene, you're also bound to take care of her afterwards.

Chapter 5: Outside the Dungeon: Getting Started

Now that you have a pretty good idea of how the Dom role works, the next step is to find the BDSM community that will help you expand your knowledge on the subject and indulge your kinky desires. Now, there are several ways to get started on this:

Finding a Partner

If you're lucky enough to have a partner who is also into BDSM, then there should be no need to seek out the BDSM community in your area. You and your partner may enjoy the relationship without question, allowing yourselves to play any scene you wish when it comes to BDSM.

Some Doms like to post advertisements through websites like Craigslist or perhaps internet communities specially set up for the BDSM scene. Although this is certainly a possibility, do not keep your hopes up that a sub will respond, especially if the setup is in your house. This is because as already mentioned, the Dom/sub relationship is anchored on trust. In a BDSM scene, the sub is highly vulnerable so there's very little chance the she will play with someone she only met through the internet.

BDSM Dungeons

The best way therefore to find a sub and to exercise your BDSM predilections is through Dungeons. Typically, Dungeons are paid-for facilities where you can hire either a Dom or a sub to play a scene with you. There are several advantages here including the fact that you'll be meeting with people who are in the same mindset as you. Additionally, dungeons are staffed by individuals who have a pretty good grip on the BDSM lifestyle and can provide you with the exact experience you want. In many cases, dungeons will guide you through the process, talk about how it works, and what can be expected.

The best thing about dungeons however, is that it helps you build a reputation. Once the community manages to see how well you take the role of a Dom, you'll be more welcomed into the lifestyle and subs will be more willing to play with you under different scenes. In some instances, you may find a sub to play with outside the dungeon.

Munch

Playing in dungeons or searching the internet can get you invited for your very first Munch. As already defined, a Munch is a gathering where BDSM enthusiasts meet in a public place for socialization purposes. This is a great way to be introduced to the society, allowing you to interact with people who follow the same lifestyle. Take advantage of your first Munch and ask different questions about BDSM and how you can proceed further into the lifestyle.

Dungeon versus Personal Play

The main difference between the two is that Dungeon Plays are often highly regulated. This means that actual sex or facsimiles thereof are often not allowed. Hence, penetration by the penis or any object in the vagina or anus is often disallowed. Instead, the pain and discomfort themselves are the replacement for the erotic component of the sex. Of course, this is not a general rule. Depending on your dungeon, the sex may or may not be allowed. Note though that generally speaking, sex combined with BDSM in an official dungeon would be termed prostitution, and therefore illegal.

Personal Plays however, typically have the element of sex into them. The sub and Dom may play with the intent of achieving orgasm at some point. Since there's usually a personal relationship during such plays, there is no problem as to the legal aspect of the whole thing.

National Kink Coming Out Day

If you feel like you're ready to show the world how kinky you are, then you can also participate in the National Kink Coming Out Day. This is a special event wherein individuals who happen to love BDSM and revel in the lifestyle come out and socialize with like minded individuals. You might want to check out this particular event and find out how you can get started as a member of the BDSM community.

BDSM Etiquette

Do NOT use the toys of other Doms for their subs. In fact, etiquette requires that you should NOT touch the toy of other Doms unless specifically allowed. The same holds true for your toys. Also note that having your own toys, whether you play in a dungeon or not is important, especially if you play with only one sub. This is for the interest of safety and health security as bodily fluids can often come up during a scene. Washing your toys should be done after every scene.

Chapter 6: More BDSM Techniques for the Bolder Dom

Being the Dominant requires that you know a lot of techniques. Otherwise, the submissive will not writhe in fear, pain, and pleasure altogether. These elements are important in BDSM, especially if you want to play the really aggressive Dom. Here are more techniques to make your play more exciting and heart-pounding:

1. USING SEX TOYS

    - You could insert connected beads to your vagina or anus then have them pulled out.

    - Use dildos (a non-vibrating phallus) to add stimulation.

    - You could use love eggs, otherwise known as oriental eggs. These are two balls connected that you place inside the body. It is powered by battery.

    - Play with suction toys on your breasts, nipples, or genitals.

    - As a Dom, use vibrator on your sub for internal and external stimulation.

2. THROUGH BONDAGE

    - Bondage Light. You could lightly bind the body to make the sub feel he/she is really a slave.

    - Bondage Heavy, where the sub is not allowed any movement.

- Place your sub in a box or a closet.

- Bind his/her breasts.

- Put your sub in a cage and play pretend that he/she be freed if he/she does as you say.

- Affix your sub on a post, as if you're crucifying the sub.

- Bind the sub's whole body.

- Bind the sub's genitals.

- Hypnotize your sub and make him/her submit freely to you.

- Wrap your sub in leather, cotton, or whatever tickles your fantasy.

- Restrain your sub outdoors or privately.

- Show other people that you are restraining your sub. The restraint could take an hour or more, even overnight. You could even restrain your sub for days, unless the sub says a safeword.

- Suspend your sub above the ground, whether vertically or horizontally. The sub can also be suspended upside down.

3. USING BONDAGE TOYS

- Blindfolds are effective in heightening other senses in a sub other than sight.

- Place the sub in a body bag, or restrict his/her movement with a duct tape.

- Make the sub wear hoods to allow a small part of the fabric for breathing or seeing.

- Gag your partner with a ball, cloth, a bit, a dildo, or any inflatable device. Duct tapes can also be used to gag the sub.

- Use a harness for your sub. Choose from leather or rope.

- Deprive your sub of hearing by making him/her wear earplugs.

- Use a metal bondage equipment such as manacles.

- Cover your or your sub's face with a mask. It adds excitement.

- Use bondage that can be freed by a key.

- Bind the sub's ankles and arms. Use handcuffs as restraint.

- In place of leather and rope, use silk scarves to restrict the sub's body.

- Place the sub in a sleep sack to immobilize him/her.

- Put the sub in a swing or a sling. Restrict the sub's movement by connecting his/her legs to a spreader bar. Strait jackets are also quite popular nowadays.

4. THROUGH SADOMASOCHISM

- Scrape or scratch the skin of your partner. You could use your nails or any abrasive material.

- Stretch the sub's anus open. This is called anal dilation. You could also place your hand inside the sub's anus.

- Asphyxiate the sub by covering his/her face with a cloth or a thin plastic.

- Torture the sub's soles (bastinado). Beat your partner lightly or heavily. Use your arms or a paddle. You could beat any part of the body for that matter (e.g. the back, the butt, chest, breast, feet, genitals, or the face). The severity of beating depends on the slave contract, however. Make sure that you inflict the right amount of pain. The logic of BDSM is to give pain as much as pleasure.

- Bite your partner. Nibble on the skin until there are red marks. This is also a method of branding, though the marks will not be permanent.

- Stretch or milk the breast. You could also do breast torture or breast whipping.

- Choke your partner, but not to the extent that he/she loses oxygen entirely.

- Use electricity to create pain or sensation.

- Slap the submissive's face. This is better done when the sub is feeling so much pleasure already.

- Use fire and heat to increase sexual sensations.

- Pull the hair of your sub. Pinch the skin, or punch a body part.

- Give your partner a scar that he/she will always remember you by. The more personal the scar, the better it is.

- Scratch the skin of your partner especially when both of you are enjoying the sexual act. Spank the sub, whether the sub is on hands and knee. Spanking can be hard or soft.

- Deliberately stretch the vagina of your submissive, or do vaginal fisting (place your hand inside her).

- If the sub is female, make her wear a bodice or a corset and tighten it. While in the act, her breasts will bulge and there will be pain. Say that you'll release the hold on the bodice if the sub is willing to be "a good girl".

There are other methods, but these are already within vanilla sex, and may not be considered BDSM techniques. A word of caution: Always make sure that your partner consents to the act. You don't want to be labeled "unsafe".

BDSM is all about entertainment. Whether you want to inflict pain or not, the bottom line is that both you and your partner should benefit from the sexual activity. After all, BDSM was meant for play, not for abuse. Whatever happens in the dungeon should stimulate you and your sub. A real Dom is in control of the play, while beginners simply experiment without any thoughts of aftercare.

BDSM is also not just about physical play. There is also mental play here. The most important thing as the Dom is that you and your sub know who's in charge in the dungeon. The switch will be good for both sexes, and there would be no struggle for power. There is only surrender.

Chapter 7: Qualities of a Dominant

In order to be a dominant , you are going to make sure that you exhibit some very important qualities that are going to determine if you are successful or not when it comes to being dominant . If you cannot show all of these qualities, you may end up being a dominant that does not have a submissive, or you are going to become a dominant that is in a relationship that many people are not going to want to be with.

Self-control

If you are not able to control yourself such as your emotions, then you are not going to be able to control that in another person. Other dominant s are going to see you as weak and too self-indulgent therefore you are not going to have the skills necessary to control how someone else is going to react emotionally. It does not matter how good your submissive is, there are going to be times that they are going to act out and resist your control. However, how you deal with that resistance is going to be what is going to encourage your submissive to give you good behavior or is going to encourage that bad behavior. The better that you can deal with their emotional outbursts, the better they are going to be as well as the happier they are because you are able to read their emotions and know what is going on and how to react to it before it gets out of hand.

A lot of the time, the problem that brings out anger or any other negative emotion is going to be that your submissive has a problem submitting and you are going to have to work that out of them. Having self-control means that you are going to be able to react to the outbursts of your submissive in a controlled manner instead of overreacting and possibly damaging your relationship with your submissive. Together you can work on a plan that is going to discourage negative behavior.

Stubbornness and emotional resilience

When you are a dominant , you are going to have to be able to create a relationship with your submissive that is going to make it to where you get what you want without having to push your submissive to a point where you damage your relationship with them. Being stubborn can be a good trait, however you do not want to push it too far or else you are going end up coming off like a child who is throwing a fit that they did not get their way. Remember that any resistance that you are met with is going to be because the submissive is having a problem with submitting. Just like was discussed in the self-control section, you are going to want to be able to control your emotions so that you are not having an outburst each time that your submissive does something that you do not like. Instead, relish in the resistance that you come up against and let it enhance your control over your submissive.

Responsibility

As a dominant you are responsible for not only yourself, but for someone else. You have to be able to have enough responsibility to know that when you are participating in play, you are not only thinking about yourself. It is in these times that your submissive is going to get harmed. You need to make sure that you are putting your submissive first because in the end, it is the submissive that has the true power to say when everything is going to stop.

Whenever you speak and come to realize that you are angry, you need to be sure that you are thinking before you speak. What you do is going to affect your submissive as well as yourself. There are going to be things that you are going to encounter that are only going to come from you because you are going to be the one who is in control of the boat that you are riding on. You have to realize that you are the one who is calling the shots and no one else.

Maturity

Once again, you are in charge of another human being. What happens to them is going to be based solely on what you decide to do. So, when something goes wrong, you cannot blame what happened on someone else. You have to step up and take responsibility for the things that you do wrong and make it right. Having power over someone else is going to make it difficult to achieve your goals and it is going to take a while for you to actual achieve the relationship that you are wanting to have with your submissive.

Being mature means that you are going to be able to be an example that your submissive can look up to and be proud of. In a dominant the submissive is going to find strength and support all of the time not just when it is convenient for him. Also, being mature means that you are going to recognize that life happens and that he cannot control everything.

You should never learn this by experimenting on your submissive! This should be something that you learn elsewhere where you are not having complete control over someone's life.

Trustworthiness

Your submissive needs to be able to put their complete trust in you. You are going to doing things to your submissive that they are not going to allow another living soul to do and if they cannot trust you completely, then how are they going to trust that you are not going to harm them?

Not only does your submissive need to be able to trust you with their body, but they also need to be able to trust you with their emotions as well. They have to know that they are going to be able to come to you with any problem that they may have and you are not going to push them away or reject them in anyway.

What does not seem like a big deal to you may be earth shattering for someone else. So, when your submissive comes to you with a problem, they have to know that you are not only going to keep it to yourself, but you are going to do everything in your power to fix it for them.

Experience and knowledge

You need to know what you are doing! There are some dominant s out there that start out as a dominant because they want to know what they are putting someone else through. While this is not going to be a requirement, it is a good place to start for some because they do not know exactly what it is that they are getting into.

You should never stop learning either. You need to keep up to date on all the information that you can possibly find so that you are not doing something that is frowned upon in the BDSM community if you participate in it.

Besides, it is a good idea to have some firm data to fall back on when you are doubting yourself. And, do not overthink things. It takes a long time to be able to know how to control someone and how that type of relationship is going to work.

Do not be afraid to ask for a mentor in the BDSM community. Having someone who is out there for you to pick their brain or ask questions when things start going south is helpful and will assist you when it comes to making sure that you are doing things the right way.

Desire

The sad thing about some people is that they are fine with someone else for short periods of time, but when it comes to being around someone all the time, they have no idea what to do to keep the relationship going.

Being a dominant is not always about controlling the other person and having sex with them all the time. You have to actually get to know the other person. You are spending considerable amounts of time with this person and you are going to want to know all that you can about them.

The more that you know, the easier it is going to be to understand what they are going through and you are also going to know when something is wrong even when they do not say anything.

Chapter 8: Rules for a Dom

When you are a dominant , there are things that you are going to want to keep in mind as you go about your life. Being a dominant is not something that you can just turn off and turn back on when the situation is right. It is something that you are going to have to experience every day of your life. You have to think of your submissive in everything that you do because whether you know it or not, what you decide to do is going to affect them in one way or another.

1. Safety has to be your top priority. This does not just mean that you have to worry about their physical safety but their emotional safety as well. It does not mean that you are the one who is harming them. Sometimes they harm themselves and you have to protect them from themselves as well as other people. If you see that there is something that is harming them, you need to make sure that you are protecting them so that it does not continue to happen.

2. Communication. Sometimes people forget that communicating is key. But, in a BDSM relationship, you have to be able to communicate. The submissive needs to feel like they are able to come to you about their needs, what they want to try, and even what they may be concerned about. The same should go for you. You do not need to be giving yourself up just to make your submissive happy. Dominant , submissive relationships are a give and take on both ends.

3. Trust your submissive or else your submissive is going to start to push you away. Why should they keep trying if all they feel they are doing is failing you? You should be able to trust your

partner until they show you that you cannot. And that goes the other way as well. Your partner needs to

be able trust you completely.

4. Whenever punishment is being administered when you are angry. If you are angry when punishment comes to from you, it should be in a loving manner and not because you cannot control your anger. If you are not able to control your anger, that is when you need to walk away and deal with it later. Be sure that you explain why you acted the way that you did. And, if you do end up finding that you punish when you are angry, you stand up and claim what you did and apologize. Then you need to make it right so that your submissive does not think that this is going to happen all of the time. Also, you should explain what it is that you are expecting out of your submissive in the future when it comes to that situation.

5. Do not be afraid to admit that you have made a mistake. You are human. However, you do not need to keep going without acknowledging that you have made a mistake or that you are blaming it on someone else. your relationship is going to continue to grow by admitting that you have made a mistake.

6. Encourage your submissive. Help her grow and do not tell her that she cannot do what she wants to do. If she has dreams, push her towards them. Your goal is to make sure that she is not staying still in life because she is not allowing you to stay static so, why should she? The more that you grow together, the better your relationship is going to be.

7. You do not know it all! Never assume that you know everything because there are always things that you are going to be able to

learn. Pick up books and read them to stay up to date on the most recent information. Read articles, and as we said earlier, do not be afraid to get a mentor.

8. Make sure that your submissive has no questions about your boundaries. You cannot just go make new rules whenever you feel like you should punish your submissive. Make sure that they know where the lines are and that if they cross them, then they are going to be punished for doing something that they know not to do.

9. Be sure to tell your submissive that you value her. You may not love your submissive like a husband loves a wife, and no one is expecting that of you. However, your submissive is doing something for you and giving up a big part of their life, so value your submissive and do not only tell her, but show her!

10. Never abandon your submissive. If there comes a time that you think that your relationship with your submissive has to end, be sure that you talk to them about it. Up until the relationship is terminated, you are responsible for your submissives emotional state.

Chapter 9: Signs of Someone Who is a Non-Dominant

There are some people that are going to act as if they are dominant s and they tend to get people hurt because they are doing something that they have no need to be doing because they do not have the proper knowledge that is going to ensure that they are not going to harm someone.

Sometimes it is hard to tell a true dominant from someone who is just playing. Even as another dominant , you need to be able to find those that are imposters because they can end up harming someone and you are going to feel like it is your fault that you did not do something when you could have.

1. While control is part of a dominant and submissive relationship, the control that a non-dominant exhibits is not going to be because it is part of the relationship. Instead, it is because they feel like they are going to lose their partner and if they are not controlling, they are going to walk out and be alone. There are a few things that they do in order to control their partner to ensure that they are not going to be able to go anywhere.

    a. They show jealousy that is well beyond what it needs to be. A little jealousy is normal, but there is a line and someone who is not a true dominant is going to cross this line.

    b. The submissive is going to be isolated from their friends and family. This is going to take a little bit of time doing but eventually they are not going to talk to any of their family or friends because they are going to feel like they will be punished if they do. This is one way that the non-dominant makes sure that the submissive cannot leave because they have nowhere to go.

    c. Social interactions do not happen without the dominant being there. This is because the dominant thinks that a simple interaction such as ordering food at a restaurant is going to come off as flirting and thus will start a relationship with that person which gives the submissive somewhere to go.

    d. When a submissive shows that they are able to do something for themselves, someone who is not a dominant is going to discourage that because once the submissive is able to do something that not only pushes themselves forward, but could end up getting them out of the relationship, the dominant is going to be left alone.

2. Their temper is explosive. The littlest thing will set a non-dominant off. This can be as simple as the wrong word being spoken or something major like a decision being made that should have been a group decision.

3. Whenever a non-dominant does not get their way, they are going to throw a temper tantrum. This is because they believe that they are supposed to always get their way because they are the ones that are in control and no one else should be able to get what they want until the non-dominant gets what they want.

4. Drugs and alcohol are usually abused and this can lead to some of the explosive behavior that is seen.

5. Whenever mistakes are made, the non-dominant is going to not take responsibility for their own actions. Instead, he is going to blame whoever is most convenient at the time.

6. Other unhealthy behavior choices are going to be made in order to make sure that the submissive is going to be kept under his thumb. This can be any number of things that can be considered abuse in a relationship.

    a. Withdrawal of affection or emotional withdrawal. In order to get their way, they are going to do the silent treatment or refuse to give their submissive intimacy so that the submissive is fearful that the relationship is going to end.

    b. Emotional blackmail. When the submissive is scared that if they do not give into what the non-dominant wants, then they are going to do whatever it is that the non-dominant wants. This is also a way for the submissive to try and make sure that the black mail that the non-dominant is holding does not get out to anyone else.

A non-dominant is going to be really good at making others believe that he is a true dominant, but you have to keep an eye on the warning signs. The first person who is going to be able to tell you about the warning signs is the submissive. However, you do not need to overstep your bounds being that it is not your submissive as well as the fact that they may be scared to speak up and save themselves.

Conclusion

Other than the rules when it comes to safety, there are no defined limits as to the practice of BDSM. The only requirements are that they are sane, safe, and consensual as originally talked about in the previous Chapter. As a Dom, here's what you should keep in mind before, during, and after a play:

- Always ask the sub what they're willing and not willing to do

- Always ask for consent

- Always exercise self control

- Always practice aftercare

BDSM is a unique community filled with people from all sides of the community. You might be surprised, but the truth is that some members come from the higher ranks of society who simply have very different preferences in their lifestyle. As long as it does not cause harm to anyone else, BDSM is a perfectly acceptable way of life.

The next step is to apply these tips and strategies to bring your sex life and your relationship to exhilarating heights.

Lastly, remember that sex is meant to be an extraordinary experience, so don't be afraid of exploring activities and sensations that are beyond the ordinary. Each of us has our own fetishes and fantasies. Are you brave enough to live out yours?

Marriage Games

Turn Your Bedroom Into A BDSM Dungeon

Introduction

If you're in a relationship with someone, it's important to keep in mind that you shouldn't be lazy in your relationship. What this means is that you have to always be adventurous, especially when it comes to having consensual sex.

How could you be adventurous then? Well, by trying BDSM, of course!

You see, BDSM is not a way to punish—but rather to involve, and to experience something that can bring you two together. BDSM can turn you into a master and a slave; a teacher and a student; a boss and his secretary—and so much more! It's like entering a different world where you can explore your sexuality even more, and be stronger as a couple. By banning inhibitions and playing different roles, a couple gets to be more in tune with each other, and gets to understand what makes each partner tick. These BDSM scenarios also allow couples to develop a better sense of trust for each other.

With the help of this book, you'll learn about 39 different BDSM roles that you can play—some for beginners, some for experienced ones, and some for experts. Risk level is also given so you'll know exactly what to expect. Generally, men act as dominants—but take note that you can always reverse roles—do what you want to.

Chapter 1: Role Plays for Beginners

1. Teach Me, Sir
Risk Level: Low

Dominant: In this role play, the dominant acts like a teacher who asked his student to come to his house for a "special project" because she's been having failing grades. Set up some books inside the room, and maybe even a board just to give it the "classroom feel". The dominant then asks the student to bend over the bed so he could spank her a bit before doing what he wants to do with her. In the end, he would tell her that she did a good job.

Submissive: The submissive enters the room, feeling ashamed of herself because of her "failing grades". She then does what the dominant has asked her to do. It would also be better to wear a white blouse and short, plaid skirt to give the illusion of being a student. She would also say sorry to her teacher for her bad grades, and would promise to be a better student, and she'd start by doing what's asked of her.

2. Aye, Aye, Captain
Risk Level: Medium

Dominant: In this scenario, the dominant would act like a captain of a pirate ship—so it would be great to wear a bandana and an eyepatch. A fake sword would also come in handy. He will come crashing through the door of a room, intended to be the submissive's lair. He'll pretend to catch her, like he wants to kidnap her, and then he'd rip her clothing before pinning her to the wall. He will then tell her that he'll do whatever he wants to her, and would do so until he's satisfied.

Submissive: The submissive will stay inside a room, preferably wearing an off-shoulder dress, and would be surprised when the dominant comes in. She'll pretend to struggle, but would allow the captain to do what he wants with her.

3. Whatever He Wants
Risk Level: Medium

Dominant: The dominant stuffs a bag and fills it up with a blindfold, wrist cuffs, ankle cuffs, and other toys, and sets it near the bedroom door. He then puts a note outside the bag telling the submissive to strip and take whatever's in the bag inside the room. If the bag contains a blindfold, write that she has to put it on, and to come inside the room. Once there, the dominant does not call her by her name, and does not reveal who he is to her—which adds mystery to the evening. He then tells her that she has to abide by what he wants to do, and she agrees.

Submissive: The submissive complies with what's written on the note, and enters the room. She'd ask the dominant what his name is, but he wouldn't reveal it to her. She then agrees to what he wants to do.

4. The Photo Shoot
Risk Level: High

Dominant: The dominant acts as a photographer who specializes in sexy, sensual photography. The dominant tells the submissive that he won't accept monetary payment for his services. He then reveals that he wants sexual favors in return, because he has photographed the submissive the way she wants. He then does what he wants to do with her, without her "knowing" (but of course, she would have to know) that he's taking a video of her. He then gives her the video in exchange for her "services".

Submissive: The submissive acts as a client who commissions a photographer to take sensual photos of her. In return, she agrees to give him sexual favors as a fee.

5. Taking the Submissive Out
Risk Level: Medium

Dominant: The dominant will pretend to take his "submissive" out. For this, he could take his submissive out to dinner and a movie, but the catch is that the submissive shouldn't speak throughout the night. He will then whisper things to her, like what he'll do to her later in the evening. At home or at the hotel, he will then tell her that she did a good job—and he'll do what he wants with her. He would also tell her certain things that she has to do for the night, such as going to the powder room and removing her underwear, or sending her a text message while her phone is in her panties—and on vibrate, just to test her. It's a good way of tempting her and letting a sexy vibe envelop them both.

Submissive: The submissive will try to be quiet the whole evening, and do as she's told. If she "disobeys", she has to be ready for "punishment" once they're home or at the hotel—or wherever they're spending the night at.

6. The Guard and the Subject
Risk Level: Medium

Dominant: The dominant pretends that he's a security guard who heard that there was a woman who's creating havoc in the neighborhood. When the guard finds the woman (the submissive), he'll bring her to the interrogation room and does a humiliating strip search on her. The dominant then asks the submissive to touch herself just to make sure she's not hiding anything else on her body—in any way.

Not satisfied, the guard tells the submissive that he'll lock her up, but then tells her that she could spend the night free if she allows him to do whatever he wants. The guard could also put it all on videotape—as evidence—in case the subject decides to tell others about what they've done in the night.

Submissive: The submissive is someone who has wrecked havoc in the neighborhood in any way possible. When the guard sees her, she tries to break free but he ultimately catches her, and she's subjected to a humiliating interrogation. She begs him to let her go, but he tells her that if she doesn't agree to giving him sexual favors, he'd have to lock her up. She then agrees to do what he wants, and "begs" him not to videotape her—but cannot do anything but agree.

7. The Punishment
Risk Level: High

Dominant: The dominant and the submissive are having fun at home, possibly watching TV, and eating some chips when they begin petting and necking. The dominant wants to do more but he then begins to see that the submissive is hesitant. After trying to ask her lightly to do more, he loses his patience and then ties her around a chair and then spanks or whips her a bit and does what he wants with her until she says sorry and begs for release.

Submissive: The submissive isn't in the mood to do a lot in bed and pushes the dominant to his limit. She ends up being tied up in a chair and allows him to have his way with her until she says sorry and asks him to release her.

8. The Thief
Risk Level: High

Dominant: The dominant enters the room looking like a burglar. He then tells the submissive to keep quiet or he'd have no choice but to hurt her. He'll then start looking for something in her drawers or closet and gets mad when he couldn't find whatever it is that he's looking for. He then charges towards the submissive and cuts her clothes off. He tells her that he'd just have her instead, and proceeds to do what he wants with her.

Submissive: The submissive is having a quiet night in her room when suddenly, a thief appears, trying to look for a certain item in the room. She tells him to go away or she'll call the police, but he takes her phone away from her. She tries to shout but he threatens her, and she ends up pleading for him to spare her life when she sees that he couldn't find whatever it is that he's looking for. She gives her body to him and lets him do what he wants with her. She even thanks him for sparing her life.

9. She's the Prize
Risk Level: High

Dominant: The dominant goes inside a room where the submissive—this time playing the role of a stripper—is standing in the corner. He then makes his way towards the submissive and tries to inspect her body a bit. He could be as creative or demeaning as possible. He would then tell her that he won a prize from the raffle at the "bar" earlier, and that she is his prize. He then ties her up, and teases her, and then uses her as his "sex toy" for the evening. He then tells her that if she disobeys, she'll be punished and she would not like it. He would really take advantage of her as his prize.

Submissive: The submissive dresses up like a stripper—or at least, someone working for a bar. She wears a corset, some stockings, and gloves and waits in a corner of the room. When the dominant comes, she learns that she's his prize for the evening, and has no choice but to give in to what the dominant asks her to do.

10. Boss and Secretary
Risk Level: Medium

Dominant: The dominant enters his "office" (turn a room of the house into a makeshift office, or if your office is "free", you can try doing it there just for a bit of fun) and when he sees his secretary, he tells her that he's had a bad day. He notices that she's lost in work so he tells her to stand up and come towards him. He then forcibly kisses her and pulls her so she could sit on the desk. He then tells him that as her boss, he has the right to her body—and she has to give in to his wishes. He then tells her to wrap her arms and legs around him and she complies. He does some foreplay on the desk and then proceeds to have sex with her on the floor before telling her to dress up as fast as she could. He then hurriedly leaves the room.

Submissive: The submissive is just patiently doing her work at the office when she hears her boss talk about how bad his day was. Secretly, she has a crush on him so when he tells her to stand up and forcibly kisses her, she gets positively jolted inside. She then does as she's told, even though she's scared that they'd be caught because she secretly wants to do it, too-and has wanted for quite a while.

11. The Proposition
Risk Level: Low

Dominant: In this scenario, the dominant acts like a lawyer who has a proposition for his young client who is involved in a drug-related crime. He notices that she's been crying too much, and he tells her that she should stop crying and listen to him instead. He then tells her that if she wants to be saved, and not go through any trials whatsoever, she should willingly agree to what he wants to happen or else he won't be her lawyer anymore. He then asks her to strip and decides what he wants to do with her, repeatedly telling her to stop crying.

Submissive: After being involved in a high-risk crime, the submissive seeks the help of a lawyer. She cries after being so desperate to get help, and then hears the lawyer saying that if she wants his help, she should strip for her and do what she wants. She feels afraid at first, but feels like she has no choice, so she does what he wants.

12. Who's Your Daddy?
Risk Level: Medium

Dominant: This is such a classic, so the dominant would be acting as if he's the submissive's "daddy". He'll enter the submissive's bedroom at night and would tell the "little girl" to keep quiet so mommy wouldn't hear. He would then tell her to get on all fours on the bed, and tell her she's been a bad girl who deserves some spanking. He would then spank her before asking her "*Who's your daddy?*" - And would then proceed to have his way with her. At the end of the night, he would tell her to keep her mouth shut so "mommy" wouldn't know about it. This is an exciting scenario to play and that's why it's the favorite of many.

Submissive: The submissive would dress up in clothes reminiscent to what a little girl would wear. If her hair's long enough, she'd have them in pigtails, too. She would pretend to be sleeping in her room when suddenly, the dominant AKA "daddy" comes in. She would ask him what's she's doing in her room and he would tell her to keep quiet. She would then ask him what needs to be done, and "pretends" to be scared when he tells her that she needs to be spanked. He tells her to follow what he orders or else, she will be punished. She then agrees and says that she won't tell "mommy" about what's about to happen. After the incident, she would bid "daddy" goodnight and would tell him that she'd always be a good girl.

13. Her Best Friend's Father
Risk Level: Low

Dominant: The dominant suits up to look like he's a grown, adult man, most specifically the father of her "daughter's best friend". He would then arrive at home to find the submissive apparently waiting for his daughter, and tells her that his daughter is not home yet, but maybe she wants to check out the big library they have? They'd then go to the library and there, he tells the submissive that he always found her to be beautiful. He then kisses her and when he hears her refuse at first, he tells her he's always known that she wants to get together with him, too. He then rips her clothes apart and begins to have his way with her. In the end, he suits up once again and tells her that he'll see her again soon.

Submissive: The submissive goes to her "friend's house" in hopes to see her, but then she only finds her friend's father. She always secretly liked her best friend's father so when he invites her to go to the library with him, she agrees and becomes secretly thrilled when he kisses her. She then tells him that she's "scared" because she's a virgin, but then he proceeds to have his way with her. She tries to be reluctant at first but also gives in and tells him that she'll also see him again soon.

14. The Prize
Risk level: low

Dominant: you win a session with a single stripper to do whatever it is that you want to them.

Submissive: you work in a strip club that allows for the clients to do whatever it is that they want. Therefore, you are going to be the perfect sex toy for your client no matter what it is that they want.

15. Photo Shoot
Risk level: low

Dominant: you are a professional photographer who has been hired by a someone to do some erotic photos. However, whenever you are done with the photo shoot, you are going to ask for payment in the form of the client becoming the plaything for you. If you so desire, you can take photos the second time around so that you have some extra keepsakes.

Submissive: you will model however the photographer asks of you and when they tell you how it is that they are requiring payment, then you are to do it without question. Even if that means that they are going to take photos of it.

16. A Night on the Town
Risk level: low

Dominant: you are going to plan a fun night out with your significant other. Make sure that they understand that you are the one in charge and that you are to be listened to no matter what is going on. Nothing is going to happen that is going to give it away because the key to the whole scenario is to make sure that no one else knows what else is going on. You can tell your submissive that you want them to go to the bathroom and remove her underpants. Or, you can tease her in a movie theater, however, you are not going to allow her to find her orgasm. Just make sure that you are keeping your play quiet.

Submissive: you are your dominate's date and you are going to do whatever it is that they order you to do. Your whole purpose is for you to keep quiet and obey so that no one knows what is going on. If someone finds out what you are doing, you are going to have to live with the embarrassment and possibly any other consequences that may come with being caught.

17. Switch tease
Risk level: low

Dominant: you are a victim who has been tied up and blindfolded. You are going to listen to her change into something that is going to drive you absolutely wild. Once she has done that, she will take your blindfold off and tease you with her body but not allow you to touch her because you are tied up. Eventually she is going to make a mistake and you are going to get free. At the point in time that you get free, you will tie her down and tease her by stripping over her and touching on her body or your body not allowing her to touch you in return.

Submissive: once you have tied your victim down and changed without him hearing you, you are going to tease him with your body by touching yourself or rubbing against his body until you slip up and he ends up getting free. Now with you being the one who is tied down, you are going to enjoy the same teasing in return.

Note: you can add in toys to your play or just leave it at bondage play.

Chapter 2: Role Plays for Experienced Couples

18. The Interrogation
Risk Level: High

Dominant: The dominant plays the role of an interrogator who has been given the chance to question a woman who's involved in a crime of some sorts. He then brings the woman to a darkened room and straps her to a chair. He then grabs her by the hair and tells her that if she does not tell the truth, she would be punished. He would then proceed to ask her questions and when she does not answer them properly, he would "punish" her by putting clothespins on her nipples and tugging on them, putting a suction cup on her clit, and spanking or slapping her on the face. When she could not take it anymore, he would tell her that he'd let her out only if she agrees to have sex with him, and she does. In the end he asks her to put her clothes back on and tells her to go because he'll be handling her case.

Submissive: The submissive wears sexy lingerie and gets put in a darkened room. She asks the interrogator to please stop what he's doing, but he just slaps her on the face and straps her to a chair. She begs him to spare her from whatever he has planned, but then interrogates her and when she can't tell him what he wants to hear, she would accept his punishments. Pleading for her life, she would ask him to please let her out in exchange for whatever it is that he wants to happen. She then hears him say that he wants to have sex with her and she agrees. Afterwards, she gets asked to leave the room. She does, and feels humiliated but thankful at the same time.

19. The Virgin Bride and the Groom's Surprise
Risk Level: High

Dominant: The dominant prepares the "honeymoon suite" by putting rose petals on the bed and on the floor. He could also dim the lights and diffuse some rose or lavender oil in the room, just so it would be a more romantic setting. After all, it's their honeymoon—but there's a catch. He still has not told his new bride that he's actually into BDSM, and then proceeds to open up a closet door (or show a box or a bag filled with toys) once she enters the room. He then tells her that as his bride, he would want them to explore this world—the world he's been living in for so long. He would then remove her gown and tie her to the bed and would also blindfold her, for extra effect. He would then use various tools on her—such as vibrators, clamps, and whips, and would tell her that she'll be punished if she comes before her time. He would then play with her until she's ready to explode.

Submissive: The submissive enters the honeymoon room, doe-eyed and scared because she's still a "virgin". She thought it was just going to be one romantic evening when suddenly, her groom shows her his collection of BDSM toys. She would then express fears because she still has not experienced any of these before. He then tells her that this is their world now, so she agrees to be tied up and to have him try the various toys on her. Whenever she feels like she's about to come, he would punish her, so she tries to hold it all in until she's really about to explode!

20. The Mermaid
Risk Level: High

Dominant: The dominant brings home a "mermaid" that he found at sea. It would be good to have an inflatable pool or a basin that could be placed in the car, together with the "mermaid". She would be gagged or taped on the mouth so she couldn't make any noise and he'd then bring her to the bathroom, and place her in the tub. He would be gone for a while and when he comes back, he would be surprised to find that her tail has come off and that she's human now. He would then proceed to play with her by using a vibrator and clamps, and would proceed to have his way with her.

Submissive: The submissive would pretend to be a mermaid—so a tail has to be around, and would be "kidnapped" by the dominant. Once she's in the tub, magic happens and she loses her tail. She would then agree to whatever the dominant wants, thinking that he's actually her savior when really, he just wants to have his way with her.

21. The Director and the Star
Risk Level: Medium

Dominant: The dominant would act like a director of a TV show or a music video, so he'd take videos of the submissive. At the end of the shoot, he would tell her that he knows she's been cheating on her boyfriend so if she does not agree to shoot a "porn" video with him, he would tell her boyfriend about it, and would even tell him that she's cheating on him with the director himself. He would then shoot her on different angles, and would even take a video of her as she performs oral sex on him. Then, he would take a video of them having sex and would tell her that he would put out this tape if she ever talks about it to anyone. He then tells her to go home for they'd have another long day tomorrow.

Submissive: The submissive goes to work to shoot for a music video or television show. When she begins to dress up for work, the director stops her and tells her that he knows she's been cheating on her boyfriend. She's shocked that he knows this and asks him what he wants so he'd keep quiet. She then proceeds to give him sexual favors and allows him to take a video of those favors and agrees that she would not talk about it to anyone.

22. The Hostage
Risk Level: High

Dominant: The dominant acts like a hostage taker who's waiting for the victim on one side of the street—for example, the garage. As the "victim" gets out of the house, he would accost her by putting a handkerchief over her mouth and bringing her inside the car. He would then bring her inside the room and restrain her by tying her up (you can do this on the bed, on the chair, or if you can put ties on the ceiling, do that, too), and would taunt her by saying she'd never be able to get out of there anymore. He would then rip her clothes apart and proceed to use various toys on her, such as a dildo, a vibrator, a whip, and clamps. He would also taunt her with degrading words and would then proceed to have his way with her. He would leave her inside the room for a couple of minutes and then would have sex with her again before locking her inside the room.

Submissive: The submissive would get out of the house not knowing someone's already waiting for her. She would then be placed inside the car then tied up in the room. She would pretend to be scared and would make lots of noise, asking the perpetrator to let her out, but of course, she would not be let out. She would then just pretend to cry as the hostage taker gets his way with her.

23. In the Dark
Risk Level: High

Dominant: The dominant would set up a dark room—it has to be really dark—where he could keep the submissive in. Then, he would go somewhere in the house where there's still light and "abduct" the submissive. He would then place her in the dark room, and ask her to eat food he's placed on the floor. When she refuses to eat—and of course, she would—he ties her up (you can strap her on a chair, or just choose to bind her while she's sitting on the floor), and throw some water on her. After doing that, the dominant would then grab her by the hair and would "force" her to perform oral sex on him. Afterwards, he would use various toys on her while she's restrained and finally, unchain her to have sex with her.

Submissive: The submissive would be waiting at a certain, lit corner of the house. It would be good to wear a sundress or anything light, and then would be surprised when a man abducts her and puts her inside the dark room. She would try to get out of her restraints but of course, she would not be able to, and would just agree with whatever the dominant wants to happen. This exercise would really build trust and connection between the couple because it's done in a dark room, which means fear might be in effect, but since it's just a scenario, in the end, everything should work out for them.

24. The Debutante
Risk Level: Low

Dominant: This one is fun. Basically, the dominant is an older guy that the submissive met at a party. It's the debutante's ball that night and her parents do not know about this guy yet. What the dominant would do is send the "debutante" messages throughout the night. After the "party", the debutante would go up to her room and would be surprised to find the dominant hiding there. He would tell her that he has a surprise for her and proceeds to tie her on the bed. He would tell her not to be scared and then proceeds to have his way with her. He then cuts off her ties and gets out of the house through the window (if possible), leaving her bewildered.

Submissive: The submissive would be surprised to receive messages from this guy she met a few days ago during her debut party. After her party, she makes her way to her room, preparing to rest, but is then surprised when she sees this guy in her room, saying that he has a surprise for her. She tells him that her parents are just downstairs but he tells her that she should not be scared. She then allows him to tie her up in bed, although she's somewhat scared, and allows him to have his way with her. She also gets a bit scared when he cuts off the ties he used on her and gets out of her room through the window.

25. The Stalker
Risk Level: Medium

Dominant: The dominant pretends to be a stalker who would text his "victim" all throughout the night. He would tell her that he has always liked her, and that she's always on his mind. He would also tell her that he's always wanted to do something to her, and with her. Bummed that he's "not getting any replies", he decides to follow her home from work (if you have a car and can really follow her home from work—with her knowledge, of course—it would be better) and then grabs her when she finally reaches home (make sure not to let the neighbors know, of course! You wouldn't want to cause a scene) and then restrain her before bringing her to her room. Once there, he would slap her and tell her that she's been a bad girl and that all he wants is to be with her. He then slaps her as he begins to touch here all over, and then leaves her tied up in bed. He then sends her one last text, saying thank you for the night and that maybe, he'd see her again sometime.

Submissive: The submissive would go home after another tiring day at work and would be surprised to receive so many messages from this stalker she's been hiding from for so long already. She didn't know that today would be the day that he finally gets to accost her, and cries for help when he restrains her on the way to her room. She tries to repulse him—but she really couldn't—and so just allows him to have his way with her. After getting what he wants, he texts her to say thank you and leaves her alone in her room.

26. The Runaway Bride
Risk Level: High

Dominant: The dominant is home when suddenly, he hears a plea from outside his door (it could just be the bedroom door so neighbors would not think you're causing a scene) and is surprised when he finds a woman in her bridal clothes standing outside the door, asking for help. He hears the woman say that she has nowhere to go and she does not want to wed his groom because she really does not love him. He then tells her to come in and then gets a pair of scissors. He suddenly rips her clothes apart. He tells the bride not to make a sound and then proceeds to tie her up in a char. He then interrogates her as to why she left his groom and tells her that she should be ashamed of herself for what she's done. He then punishes her by clamping her, and then interrogates her even more before asking her to perform oral sex on him. He then brings her to the bedroom and forces her to have sex with him before telling her she could now stay with him because no one would like her anymore. She then agrees.

Submissive: The submissive is a runaway bride who runs towards a house/room because she fled from this man whom she does not really like. She thought she would finally get the help she needs when someone opens the door, but apparently, this man is just a dominant who wants to have fun with her in exchange for her stay in the house. She is scared at first, especially because she does not know this man but is too scared to say anything so he lets him have his way with her. When he tells her that no one would want her anymore, she agrees to stay in the house with him.

27. The Cyber Couple
Risk Level: Medium

Dominant: This is a fun, exciting scenario to play. What would happen is that you would be in two separate rooms where he'd be video-chatting with his submissive. At first, it would just be fun until he brings up the idea of playing with each other online. He would then give instructions for the submissive to follow—so he could watch her touch herself, and he would do the same, too. What's good about this is that it brings up tension and it allows the couple to be more at home with themselves. He would then tell her that if she refuses, she will be punished later. Then, when they're almost about to explode, the dominant would ask the submissive to come to his room and when she does, he would punish her for what she did not follow earlier. He would then force himself on her and could even videotape the experience, too.

Submissive: The submissive is chatting with her master online when he tells her that he wants to see her touch herself. At first, she is hesitant, but then she follows. She is then asked to come to the dominant's room. Once there, she is punished for earlier transgressions, and then she allows him to have his way with her, promising that they'll do this again sometime soon.

28. The Borrowed Lady
Risk Level: High

Dominant: The dominant comes home to find this slave that he has borrowed from her master at home, waiting for him. He then asks her to kiss his manhood, and pets her as a form of greeting. He then gives her a bowl of water to drink from and she does as she's told. Then, he tells her to follow him to his room, on all fours—this might seem degrading but is actually a fun, really interesting thing to do. Once in the room, the dominant suspends the submissive above the bed and then plays with her using various toys. When he's satisfied, he proceeds to have sex with her.

Submissive: The submissive waits for the dominant inside the living room and follows whatever he asks her to do. She says thanks that he wanted to borrow her, but is punished when she says something so she learns to keep quiet. She then lets him have his way with her and thanks him after doing so.

29. The Construction Worker
Risk Level: Medium

Dominant: The dominant dresses up (or down) as a construction worker—with an oiled body and with some construction tools in tow. He has to nail some ropes to a wall and then the submissive (or the client) would be around to ask what he's doing. He would then say that she has no right to ask him that, and then proceeds to grab the client, forcibly kiss her, and tie her to where he has nailed the ropes. He would then slap her and tell her that he sees the way he looks at him all the time—and he knows she wants to be with him. He would then proceed to ravage her body and force his way on her. Then he would take off the ropes, and leave her alone, naked and spent.

Submissive: The submissive would check what her construction worker has been nailing on the walls when suddenly, he grabs and kisses her and ties her to the ropes on the wall. She's scared, but she has always had this secret crush on him so she's also thrilled about what could happen next. She lets him have his way with her until he's satisfied, and she is then left spent and naked in the room.

30. Surprise Beginnings
Risk level: Low

Dominant: While the submissive is away to work or out at another various location, the dominate needs to take a brown paper back and put in a set of restraints in it. The restraints are going to be things like ankle cuffs or even hand cuffs. The dominate can also add in a blindfold if they so desire to.

Next, the dominate is going to place this bag next to the bedroom door or the door of the house if you are so daring and then place a piece of paper with it that has a set of instructions with it. These instructions can be anything that the dominate likes such as that they cannot go through the door until they have completed the assigned task.

Submissive: When returning home, the submissive is to follow the instructions on the piece of paper to a "T" as their master desires. So, if you are to strip and place the restraints on before you are able to enter the house, then you are to strip and do as your master has ordered of you.

31. Interrogation
Risk level: High

Dominant: your job is to get the submissive to tell you the information that they know. In order to do this, you can use paddles, clothespins and even mock "rape" if that is how far it goes. What you are trying to do is to break your submissive until they break and tell you what they know and you do not. You will continue to intensify your interrogation techniques until they break.

Submissive: you will know a piece of information that your dominate does not. You are going to look at the top card in a deck of cards and not tell your dominate what that card is.

32. Pirate
Risk level: medium

Dominant: you are a pirate going through the town plundering for treasure. Whenever you reach the house of the maiden of the town, you are going to break in and wrestle with her until you take control. Swooping down, you will rip her clothes from her body and then push her against the wall. It is at that moment that you are going to make sure that she cannot move from you while you are describing in detail what it is that you will do to her. after you have done that, you are going to ravish her. If you have an eye patch and a bandanna, then that will add to the effect of you actually being a pirate.

Submissive: you are the local maiden and when the pirate comes into your home, you are going to wrestle with him but ultimately find that you are helpless and then are going to be taken by the pirate up until he is satisfied.

33. Ravishment
Risk level: medium

Note: this works great for female submissives

Dominant: you are going to enjoy a romantic evening with your significant other such as a candle lit dinner, wine in front of the fire place, anything that is romantic for you two. You are also going to make out and cuddle with your significant other but you will not get any. Several times you may get hit or pinched and then you are finally going to be fed up and tie up the submissive and have your way with her up until she is begging you for release.

Submissive: you will enjoy a romantic evening set up by your significant other and then when he keeps insisting on having sex, you will slap him or pinch him and get up to go away. Ultimately, he is going to tie you down and not allow you to have an orgasm until you are begging for it.

34. Crime and Punishment
Risk level: medium

Dominant: you are a cop and you have caught the female doing something that is against the law, you will need to frisk your criminal and then tie her hands because there are no handcuffs being that it has been a long and busy night at the station. In the event that the criminal smarts off, you are going to gag her or even spank her if that is something that you want to do.

Submissive: you can either stand at the corner of your garage in "hooker" clothing and offer up your services to him before you find out that you are talking to a vice cop. Once you have been frisked and cuffed to the bed or a chair, if you are not gagged, you can try and bribe the cop into having your body in exchange for being let go without being placed in jail.

35. Exchange of Power
Risk level: medium

Dominant: you are going to allow your submissive to have power because she has a talisman that takes away your power and gives it all to her. You are going to do whatever it is that she wants which is going to tease you and tell you what to do. You can either kiss her and it takes away all the power of the talisman or you can "punch" her and knock her out. Once she is powerless again, you are going to tie her down and have your way with her unconscious body.

Submissive: you have something that is giving you the power to be the Domme over your dominate. You can order him to do whatever it is that you want him to until he gets you to become unconscious. Once you are unconscious, you are going to be tied up and ravished. You of course are not going to be unconscious and you are going to be able to feel it all.

Note: be sure that you know each other's limits so that if you do the "punch" then you are going to know how hard to hit them so that you are not taking things too far.

36. Burglar
Risk level: medium

Note: this is good for a guy to do to a girl

Dominant: call up your significant other and convience them that there is a burglar going around her neighborhood breaking into homes that are unlocked and have women in them wearing whatever it is that you want her to be wearing. Be sure that you not only sell the breaking in story, but make it to where she cannot possibly not be in what you want her to wear and have her door unlocked.

Around that time, you are going to "break" into her house and knock her out. This can be as simple as placing a piece of cloth over her mouth that has chloroform on, but of course it is not going to be real. If you do not want to do this, you can always just have her faint because there is a strange person in her apartment. Once she is knocked out, you will take her to the bedroom and strip her down and tie her to the bed.

Ransack her room to make it more real before you take advantage of her and then leave with some of the stuff that is not valuable. You are going to want to make sure that you are wearing an outfit that does not give away who you are.

When you are escaping do not go through any door that will lock behind you. Come back in a different shirt acting as the concerned friend or lover and find her tied up and then untie her.

If you are not wanting to give her the chance to know when you are coming over, just tell her that you have been seeing news reports about break ins in her area and overpower her.

Submissive: you are going to play along with the break in allow your partner to ravage you and then be untied when he comes back. You can struggle a little if you want, however, it is up to you on how it is going to go so that both of you are comfortable with what is going on.

37. Burglar Part two
Risk level: medium

This is going to be the same as the one above, however, you are going to have the submissive be the one who is breaking in and she is breaking in to a cops home. When she is caught, the cop will tie her up and ravage her so that he does not have to take her to jail.

38. Deprogramming
Risk level: medium

Dominant: you are a person who has rescued an innocent victim from a cult that has been brainwashing its members. You are going to make the victim do things that are for your own gratification that they may not have done to themselves or that they used to do but do not anymore because of the brainwashing.

Submissive: you are going to follow orders from your deprogrammer and do whatever it is that he is asking you to do all in hopes that it is going to override the brainwashing that is coming from the cult that kidnapped you. Everything that you are going to be asked to do is going to be sexual in nature and for the deprogrammer's gratification.

Note: if you want this to be more BDSM, have your submissive do things that you normally might do, such as using a crop between her legs to make herself more sensitive or placing clamps on her nipples.

Chapter 3: Role Plays for Experts

39. The Test Subject
Risk Level: High

Dominant: The dominant would act as the lab expert who has strapped his test subject on the lab table. He would begin to kiss every part of her body and would also photograph her so he could add the photos to his important files. He would then try various objects on her, such as a vibrator, a nipple clamp (or even clothespins as clamps), and suctions. He would see how she reacts and would record it. He would then proceed to take a video of the test subject as he has his way with her body. Finally, he takes the straps off the body of the test subject and leaves her alone.

Submissive: So, what's the catch? Of course, there is, right? Well, the submissive has to have lots of patience because she wouldn't be allowed to talk (except for certain reactions when the toys are used on her) because she is a test subject. She would be "hurt" when she speaks. It's a good way of testing one's limits and just seeing how much she could do, and how much she could hold everything in. It's also a way of testing how much she tests her "master", allowing him to play with her body like that.

40. In the Cult
Risk Level: High

Dominant: The dominant has to prepare a dark room fit for the leader of a cult—with certain photos of him as a "leader", and with flowers, and a bed surrounded with candles (or lamps, or electric candles—whichever you prefer). He would then bring his submissive (a "virgin lady from the cult") inside the room and ask her to perform oral sex on him as he "blesses her". He would then undress her and tie her to the bed. After doing so, he would proceed to ravage her body. He would put clothespins on her nipples and tug on them with the use of a twine and would also perform oral sex on her, telling her not to speak. Again, control is highly important in this scenario. Afterwards, he would play with her body in any way he could, and would then enter her. He would leave her alone in bed and would return to tell her she has to get out of the room, naked and spent.

Submissive: Again, the submissive should have lots of control of herself in this scenario as she'll be the innocent, virgin lady from the cult. Wearing a white slip dress (or even a white blanket or towel wrapped around her), she would be brought to the leader's lair and she would oblige to whatever he asks of her. She would allow him to really play with her body, and wouldn't object to anything. She would also leave the room naked once he's done with her, just so the scenario would really take effect.

41. 2 Become 1
Risk Level: Medium

Dominant: Here, the dominant would act as two people who are sharing the same lady—just imagine how much fun and excitement that could bring! First, he'll act as the friend of the woman's boyfriend. He would pretend to meet her in one area of the house, and would ask her why she's still with her boyfriend. He would then take off her panties and would play with her clit and then proceed to lick her all over, letting her wear her panties and wetting them. Then, he would be waiting in the bedroom for her girlfriend (now, he's the boyfriend), and would ask her where she's been. She would not answer at first so he'll inspect her, and would notice that her panties are wet. He'd ask her whether or not she's wet for him and when she could not answer directly, he would slap her on the face and would then tie her in bed so he could have his way with her, telling her that he only belongs to her, even though he knows she's been doing it with someone else, too. The thought that there is "someone else" could actually be exciting, at least for this scenario.

Submissive: The submissive would act as the cheating girlfriend (again, you could do this vice-versa) and would have sex with her boyfriend's best friend before proceeding to come home to her boyfriend. She would then receive his punishments because she has been a bad girl and she's not "loyal" to him. This scenario is really fun and is quite a new adventure for most couples.

42. The Slave
Risk Level: High

Dominant: This is probably one of the most challenging scenarios around. Basically, the dominant would really act like a slave master. He would keep his "slave" inside a huge cage (make sure it's really huge enough to hold a person in) and would go forth with his day (or at least a few hours or minutes) before going inside the room to get his slave out. He would pull her with a twine or leather rope attached to her choker and ask her to drink from a water bowl on the floor before whipping her a bit. He would then play with her body with clothespins or clamps, and would then ask her to give him head before tying her up on the bed and having his way with her. Afterwards, he would untie her and ask her to come back to her cage, crawling, and without standing up.

Submissive: The submissive would be inside a cage, waiting for her master to come and would crawl towards him once he asks her to come. She would then give him head and do as she's told, even receiving some whips for it. After his master has had his fill of her, she would crawl back like a good pet to her cage. It may be crazy for some, but this really is one of the best master-slave scenarios you could play with.

43. The Maid and her Master
Risk Level: Medium

Dominant: The dominant would act like the tired, sexless boss who comes home one evening to find that his wife is not at home but the sexy, classic French maid is. Upon finding her in the kitchen, he would ask her to feed him not with food, but with her cunt. He would then ask her to come to the bedroom with him, and tells her that if she tells anyone about it, she would be punished and would never find a job anymore—anywhere. He then asks her to touch herself as he watches. Then he would take her clothes off and would have his way with her. Afterwards, he'd hear the bell ring and would tell her to hide in the closet, and he would then make his way outside.

Submissive: The submissive should dress up as a French maid who's doing work at home when her boss comes, telling her that he has not been properly fed by his wife in a while. She gives him head and he does the same for her and tells him that she's scared his wife might be coming home anytime soon, but then he tells her that she should just do what he wants, and she agrees. She allows him to have his way with her and then hides in the closet once they're done. The "thrill of being caught" makes this a really fun scenario to play with.

44. The Car Ride
Risk Level: Medium

Dominant: This would be a fun but challenging scenario to play with because it basically happens in the car. What would happen is he'd have this woman handcuffed to a side of the car as she plays with his manhood. He can drive around the house (if you have a large backyard), or could go around the streets—just make sure the scenario would not be too suspicious, or else you might get in trouble! The dominant could also ask the submissive to give him head or else she will be punished. Afterwards, he would bring her back inside the house, still handcuffed and would do what he wants with her.

Submissive: The submissive would be handcuffed in the car, waiting for instructions from her dominant and would do what he asks her to, knowing that she'd be punished if she doesn't. Once in the house, she would still be handcuffed as she waits for him to do whatever he wants with her. Afterwards, she would thank him for what he's done and promise to be a better girl next time.

45. In the Garden
Risk Level: High

Dominant: This one is quite challenging, and has that hint of exhibitionism. Basically, the dominant should prepare the garden by placing a bed on one side, surrounded by flowers. The bed should be filled with flowers, leaves, and petals, too, and there should be a safe tree or post where the submissive could be tied up. Or, he could also prepare a makeshift garden (probably in a room or basement of the house where he could put fake grass). Then, the dominant should lead the blindfolded submissive by pulling on her nipple clamps with twines or ropes, and then pulling her tied hands. She would then be tied to a pole or a tree and the dominant would play with her and would tease her before tying her to the bed in the middle of the garden. Again, there's a certain thrill that could be felt when people know they're about to be caught! He would then have his way with her in bed and bring her back to the house, still tied up.

Submissive: The submissive would be naked all throughout this scenario, and would really feel like she's been ravished in a garden. As she's tied up, she shouldn't make unnecessary noises—or else, the neighbors might wonder what's happening—and also to give the effect that she's really submitting to her partner. She would also allow him to bring her back in the house while still tied up, just to maximize the effect of the scene.

46. The Mile High Club
Risk Level: Medium

Dominant: Well, this doesn't necessarily have to be done in the airplane. What the dominant can do is call his submissive (who's dressed up as a stewardess) inside the bathroom—or any small space in the house—and then ask her to give him favors. When she is reluctant, the dominant would forcibly kiss her and make her feel ashamed of herself. He would then ask her to strip for him and when she disagrees, he would do it for her and would then force himself on her, even watching her dress up again after their deed as she has some "work" to do.

Submissive: The submissive would dress up as a flight attendant and would be surprised when a passenger calls her to the bathroom with him. She would repulse his actions until she couldn't anymore and would just agree to do what he wants. She would then hurriedly put her clothes back on so she could get back to her job, before they get "caught".

47. Sleeping Beauty
Risk Level: High

Dominant: This is a twisted take on the classic fairytale. Basically, the dominant finds this room where a sleeping princess is waiting to be awakened. He then comes towards her and takes pictures of her sleeping self and proceeds to slice her dress (with scissors or a knife—your choice—just be careful) and begins to kiss her. She opens her eyes and is surprised to see him, but he does not stop there. He takes out a duct tape from his pocket and tapes her before tying her hands and feet on the posts of the bed (or however way he wants). He then manages to get out certain toys and tries them on her. He teases her with a rod with a feathered end, a riding crop, some clamps, and suctions, and takes photos of her after playing with her little by little. Then he slaps her, kisses her, and begins to have his way with her. Afterwards, he takes her with him, and is now his new slave.

Submissive: The submissive is waiting to be awoken in bed by her "prince" that then turns out to be a dominant. She tries to struggle at first, but just lets the prince do what he wants with her for fear that she'll be "asleep for a long time again". It's a fun way to test one's patience and control, too—so this one is worth trying.

48. The Show of a Lifetime
Risk Level: High

Dominant: Another fun but challenging one, this one should be done late, late at night and with the lights off. What should happen is that the submissive has to be bound and gagged, and should be looking out the window. The dominant would then come in the room and remove the gag but then tell the submissive that she has such a body that the world should see. Again, when people feel like other people are going to watch them, they feel this certain thrill inside! The dominant would then play with the submissive's body for a while, not allowing her to look at him, but to just look out the window and would then cover the submissive's mouth with his hand and would have sex with her right then and there. Afterwards, he would tie her up and let her show off her body in the window. He would then go down and take a photo of her to end the night.

Submissive: The submissive would be tied up while facing a window—the couple has to agree on this and have to make sure that people won't see—and would allow her dominant to do what he wants with her.

49. The Doctor and the Patient
Risk Level: High

Dominant: Set up a makeshift clinic in the room with stethoscopes and some tools that could be used to perform a checkup on the patient. The dominant should also wear a doctor's costume, and then ask the submissive—AKA the patient—to come into the room. He would then check her up by feeling her breasts and would ask her to take her top off before taking a photo of her, presumably for his files. He would then ask her to remove her skirt or pants and would use a flashlight to see what's inside her vagina (without inserting it, of course!). He would also put clamps on her to "test" her and would say that she needs to lie down. He would then cuff her to the bed and would take more pictures before playing with her by using a riding crop and a feather duster. Afterwards, he would tell the patient that the only way to "cure" her is by allowing the doctor to use her body. He would then do what he wants with her and would ask her to get out of the "clinic" without any clothes on.

Submissive: The submissive would go to the "doctor's office" for a checkup, and would then adhere to what the doctor says because she wants to be healed. She would then allow him to have his way with her and would also walk out of the room naked, because it's what the doctor ordered.

50. The Frat Girl
Risk Level: High

Dominant: The dominant would act as the leader of a frat waiting to take his prize for the night—a girl waiting for him inside the room. He would then find a woman (the submissive, of course), spread-eagled and tied up in bed waiting for him to ravish her. He would ask her questions but she would not answer so he would be prompted to "punish" her by means of using a feather duster—or any rod with a feather at the end—to tease her. He would use it on her clit, then place clothespins on her nipples and would tug on them with a twine. When she cries, he would hurt her more, and when he's satisfied, he would then have his way with her. He could do it for a couple of times, and would leave the room with her still tied up.

Submissive: The submissive would just be waiting for the dominant to come into the room as she's tied up in bed and would be punished when she cries because her job is to satisfy the leader of the frat. Once he's done with her, she would say thank you (after he tells her to) and would stay tied up in bed.

51. The Good Wife
Risk Level: High

Dominant: Finally, the dominant could act like he's the President of the United States who wants to play with his wife. He would then call his wife and would hurriedly rip her clothes off before cuffing or tying her hands, and asking her to bend. He would then use her back as a place to put his glass of wine on, and when she budges, he would punish her by using a riding crop on her. When that's done, he'd proceed to have oral sex with her and would ask her to do the same. Finally, he would let her sit on the desk and force himself on her there, asking her to put her clothes back on and go back to their room.

Submissive: The submissive would play the role of the President's wife and would do as she's told. She needs to have loads of control to balance the wine when she's asked to, or she'd get punished. She'd also give her body to her husband, and would go back to their room once he's done with her.

52. Ghost
Risk level: Medium

There are going to be three players involved and one of these players will be a "ghost" therefore not talking and invisible to the other two players. As the dominate you are going to make out with your submissive while allowing the ghost to do whatever it is that they desire to the other two players.

These other two players are going to blame each other for what it is the ghost is doing believing it is the other person doing these things. Such as groping so on and so forth.

As the ghost, he or she is free to do whatever it is that she so wishes to do without getting any blame! This is a great role for the dominate while the two submissive are the ones making out on the couch.

53. Night Security
Risk level: High

Dominant: as the dominate you are going to be the security guard and you are going catch the submissive doing something that they are not supposed to do. You are going to catch the submissive and make a deal with them so that they do not have to go to jail. You are going to humiliate them or do whatever it is that you agree upon while it is videotaped.

Submissive: you have committed a crime and do not want to go to jail therefore, you are going to allow your dominate to do whatever it is that they are wanting to do to you on camera so that you do not go to jail. The night guard may humiliate you or molest you, however, it is all so that you do not go to jail.

54. Secret Past
Risk level: Medium

Dominant: You are from the past and you have things that could end up destroying the marriage of an ex-girlfriend. Things such as photos and videos that they may not want to come to light. What you are wanting is a favor in trade for keeping the black mail that you have secret.

Submissive: in order to save your marriage, you are going to allow the blackmailer to do whatever it is that they want no matter what their demands are. You may end up being asked to be completely exposed at your front door or anything else that the black mailer may request of you.

55. Hostage
Risk level: high

Dominant: you are going to book a room at a hotel in a 'seedy' part of the town in order to make this one feel more real. You are trying to escape the cops and you take a hostage in order to get them off your trail. You will drive too fast for the hostage to get out of the car and maybe even tie their hands together so that they cannot use them. When you get to the hotel, you are going to take the hostage into the hotel room and take advantage of their body.

Submissive: you are a hostage and you are going to have to go along for the ride with the criminal because they are driving too fast for you to escape and even if you could escape, you would end up harming yourself. So, when they get to the hotel room, you are going to be taken advantage of by the criminal.

56. Mad Scientist
Risk level: medium

Dominant: you are a mad scientist that is doing experiments on your victim. You can wear rubber gloves and a lab coat. You are going to strap your victim down a table and conduct experiments. You can hold your victim down for hours and not allow them to orgasm if that is what you are wanting. You can do whatever you want because you are testing different theories on your victim.

Submissive: you are going to be tied down to a table while the mad scientist does his experiments on you. You may not be allowed to come or you may be able to come up until you cannot physically anymore.

Note: if you are in a polyamorous relationship, you can change this to where there is a lab assistant that is the submissive and the victim is the innocent one.

57. Exorcism
Risk level: high

Dominant: you are a priest who has been called in to cast out a demon inside of a female. You are going to do everything that you can possibly think of but nothing is going to work. Eventually, you are going to be seduced into having sex with the demon.

Submissive: you are a virgin who is possessed and the demon inside of you is sexually charged up and makes you talk about yourself in very humiliating ways. Eventually, you are going to be using your body -even though your character does not know how to- and seducing the priest before having sex with him. Everything that you do with the priest is going to be coming from the demon and not your actual body.

Note: you can make this more humiliating if you want by recording it or you can add in some kinky actions where the demon touches the body that it is possessing and doing things that the normal person would not do. If you want to make it more interesting, you can say that both of you are virgins and you try to fight the seduction until in the end you end up both losing your purity.

Conclusion

I hope this book was able to help you to learn about various BDSM scenarios that you can follow and play with. The next step is to have fun! Don't be scared to try these scenarios and be in tune with your sexuality. If you consensually want to do this as a couple, then it means you're in for a good time! Try these scenarios and see what they'd do for you.

Finally, if you enjoyed this book, then I'd like to ask you for a favor, would you be kind enough to leave a review for this book on Amazon? It'd be greatly appreciated!

Thank you and good luck!

BONUS: Preview of our fiction book Taming the Tigress: A Journey To Submission

Chapter 1: Caged

Punishment

I awoke in pitch blackness. I was all alone. I waited for it to come... the dread, the panic. It didn't. At first, I thought that the cold had numbed me, body and soul. But then I remembered. And I felt the stirrings of excitement in my gut, the involuntary clench of my cunt, triggered by the remembrance of the night before.

Was it really last night that he came here? Or was it the night before that? I could scarcely remember.

In the dungeon, there were neither days nor nights. Only darkness bleeding into further darkness. I counted my days not by the mornings or the evenings. No, the Master was my universe, my rising and my setting sun. My days began with his touch. And my days died each time he left. His touch... oh I tried to remember it. I shivered in the cold and tried to recall the warmth of his hands encircling my ankles, travelling up my legs, my thighs, tracing the triangle of my pubic hair. He took his sweet time knowing fully well how he was torturing me. At this memory, lust spread like wildfire all over my body. I remembered everything with stunning precision although the occasions when he would actually touch me seemed so rare compared to the moments I spent alone in the dungeon.

I felt the ache in my stretched muscles. In the dungeon, every single inch of my body was alive with pain. Yet every fiber of my being tingled with excitement. My hands were cuffed and tied to a high pole. My legs were spread wide apart. My toes were barely touching the cold stone floor. Time trundled at a snail's pace and I spent the hours wavering between consciousness and unconsciousness, teetering between sanity and madness. I would strain my ears listening to the sounds of his footsteps, hoping he would come. There were times when I could've sworn I heard his footsteps. They were heavy, leisurely, torturous... Yet I would hear the sound stop just outside the door. I would hear the rasping sound of his breathing, sense the heat of his body from the other side. At those times, I would be tempted to call out his name, to beg him to come to me. But then I'd remember what the Master had said to me: "Not a sound, *mon chaton.*"

Ah yes, he called me his kitten. I was his pet. His strokes were always gentle. Until I misbehaved. Then he brought me to the dungeon.

Once, I dared myself to call him. Just once. Just so I could feel him near me again. When I first opened my mouth, it was as if my tongue had been severed. I tried to scream out his name but it came out as a dry croak. My throat was parched. I hadn't drunk anything in days.

He saw me, of course. I had no idea how many hours he spent looking at me from the monitor in his bedroom.

He came for me then. My Master, my Savior. A weak yellow light tiptoed into the room and I felt the familiar damp sensation spreading between my thighs. The Master carried a gas lamp in one hand and a bucket of water in the other.

He let me drink tiny sips from his open palms. I licked his palms clean, wasting not a single drop. I kept licking his palms, flicking my tongue against his hard flesh. He flipped his hand and I licked the back of it, lovingly, eagerly; perhaps a bit too eagerly because he pulled it suddenly away from me.

I looked into his eyes beseechingly. *Please, take me.* I thought, though I dared not speak the words out loud. *Please.*

He shook his head slowly. Then he walked away, leaving me sobbing in the dark. I knew then that that was my punishment for attempting to speak.

Reward

I knew that my obedience would not be for nothing. I heard his footsteps. They were quick, decisive, urgent.

The Master wanted me and he wanted me then and there.

The door swung open and I kept my gaze downward, not daring to ruin things by being too presumptuous. His breathing was heavy and I saw the bulk of his cock straining rebelliously against the fabric of his trousers. I knew my obedience had turned him on. Inside, I rejoiced. I knew I did well. I behaved and stayed put and waited for him in that dungeon. It was time for my reward.

He produced the key from his pocket and yet despite his obvious urgency, he unlocked the cuffs and untied the ropes slowly. My knees were so weak and my muscles were extremely exhausted that I fell towards him.

The Master caught me in his arms. His breath was hot in my ear as he whispered: "Lie down, Katharine."

I lay down and the coldness of the stone was cruel. It didn't matter.

"Good, my pet." he said. "Now, keep your hands on your sides."

So I did. My legs were splayed, ready to receive him. My palms flat on the floor.

The Master knelt in front of me, unzipped his trousers and freed his furious flesh.

He grabbed my ankles and raised my legs so they were pointing toward the ceiling. Then he pushed them down towards me so that my feet were on either side of my head. I became extremely aware of how exposed I was to him.

Without warning, he impaled me with a single penetrating fuck. He pierced me, flesh and soul. I screamed with pleasure and gratitude.

He moved in and out of me and with each filling thrust, his balls slapped hard against my cunt. My moist cunt involuntarily convulsed around his rigid cock and my love liquid poured generously around him.

He gasped.

I looked up to see his handsome leonine face. It was contorted in ecstasy. For a brief moment, just before he shuddered and released his hot spunk into me, I caught a glimpse of a side of him that I rarely saw.

I always wished I could freeze time, capture that image of him, and hold it forever. But right now, I am his slave. He is my Master.

How did I get here?

I *wanted* to be here, had begged to be here. I wanted to surrender my life into his hands.

Chapter 2: The Tigress

How did I get here?

It all started with an awkward incident at the ladies' room.

"The Tigress was at it again this morning." said the whiny voice that trickled from the bathroom stall. "I find it really hard to concentrate on my work when she's like literally breathing down my neck."

Laughter oozed from the other stall. "Looks like someone needs to get laid."

My first reaction was fury. Who the fuck do these bitches think they are? They work for *me*. Then I realized how pathetic that sounded. Me, bullied by my own employees. I didn't even know what their names were or what departments they're from.

The Tigress. That's what they called me. I used to think that it was a fond nickname, owing to my fierceness and my success. Until I realized that it wasn't.

I waited for the women to come out. When they did, I looked at their pale faces and said: "You're fired. Both of you."

Then I left, feeling terrible over my extreme immaturity.

"They *love* working for you." Joan, my secretary, who is also coincidentally my only friend at the office, told me. "But they also hate working for you. If that makes any sense…"

It did make sense. I was too uptight. My ill temper was contagious. Somehow, with my controlling attitude, I created a hostile work environment for my employees.

I decided to take the afternoon off and asked Joan to cancel my next two appointments.

"How did the delivery go?" I picked up my purse, ready to leave.

I was talking about the anonymous client who ordered chartreuse silk dresses by the bulk. Here's the catch: Through the past year, it was always several pieces of the exact same design, color, and size. It was weird. The money, though, was always paid up front. In fact, I owed the expansion of my little dress shop partly to that client's patronage. So I figured, if she wanted to use that single design as some sort of disposable daily uniform, then so be it.

That's not to say that I hadn't been curious. In fact, I used to be the one who personally delivered the dresses to the mansion. It was always received by different maids whose bland faces betrayed nothing. I knew that the mansion was owned by Louis Archambault as in Archambault Pharmaceuticals. But as far as I knew, there was no Mrs. Archambault.

I tried Googling him, of course. Apparently, he's a very private person. He was handsome, disturbingly so; a tall man with piercing eyes. In his photos, his lips were curled to form a curt half-smile... a cold, almost cruel curve. But I had a feeling that they could be warm and tender when he wanted them to be.
I even went so far as to send him a thank you gift: a dress of a different design. Then I got flowers and a formal thank you note, no doubt written by his secretary. After a while, I just gave up trying to find out who the gowns were for. For all I knew, they were

for him. Still, for some ridiculous reason, I kept his picture in one of my folders. I looked at it from time to time.

"They're still here." Joan's voice punctured my thoughts.

"What?"

"The gowns are still here. Winona was supposed to deliver them."

"Well, why didn't she?" I asked, starting to get irritated.

"Um, you just fired her..."

"Shit."

#

Before I could even bother to introduce myself, the new maid ushered me into the house while the other unloaded the boxes from my car. It was my first time to see the mansion's interior. It was palatial.

"You're late." she scolded.

"Oh." I said. "I know. I'm so--"

"Shush!" She cut me off, harshly. "He'll be here soon. Let's get you ready."

I hardly paid attention to what she said after that. I let her drag me up the stairs.

He'll be here soon... That was all I could think about. *Him!*

So I played along, not thinking about the consequences.

Until then, it didn't really occur to me how badly I wanted to meet him. One peek, I told myself. And then I'll come clean.

When she slipped me into one of the silk dresses, I realized that it was my size.

So, I thought. *Mr. Archambault likes his escorts in my green dresses.* And the maid mistook me for one of them. I wasn't exactly sure how I felt about that.

I was led into his office.

And there he was in all his dominant glory.

"Sit." he said sharply.

I found myself automatically dropping into a chair.

"Not there." He said again. He pressed his hand on his desk. "Here."

There was a magnetism in his voice that I couldn't resist. Without peeling my gaze from his lion-like face and without understanding myself, I sat on the edge of the table.

When his fingers dug into my shoulders, I felt the energy from his touch. The current traveled all the way from my shoulders to my clit. I pressed my legs together. I was starting to get wet.
He lifted my skirt and pried my legs open with one swift gesture. Blood rushed to my face as I realized that he was smiling at the swiftly spreading puddle of pussy juice on my panties.

I opened my mouth but my indignant protest came out as a gasp.

He had entered me with his fingers, a heavenly assault.

Then, he withdrew his hand up to his lips to taste me.

"It's nice to finally meet you, Ms. Mallory."

He flashed me his cold, cruel half-grin and for a fleeting moment, I felt fear.

Instinctively, I got to my feet and raised my hand to slap him. But he caught it and in one deft movement, he turned me over so that I was leaning facedown onto the table.

He pulled down my panties. I felt his erection pressing against my ass. I trembled with anticipation. I expected him to enter me roughly from behind.

Slap!

The ruler landed on my bum, causing the flesh to sting.

Then he ran his palm soothingly over my smarting butt cheeks.

"I do not tolerate tardiness." he said.

Slap!

The ruler came down, harder this time.

Was he *punishing* me?

I ought to have stopped him. I ought to have run away. I ought to have done a lot of things.

But I stayed.

Slap!

Tears stung my eyes.

"*Never* raise your hand against me!" he said roughly into my ear.

I heard the silk ripping away beneath his hands. My body flooded with proportionate amounts of lust and fear.

"Beautiful." he sighed. "You are a blank canvass."

But he didn't fuck me like I hoped he would.

Instead, I listened to his breath waxing and waning as he masturbated.

I tried to face him but he held my head down, my cheeks pressed hard against the table.

"Stay down." he ordered. "You are no lioness. You are my little kitten. That's all you are, *mon chaton.*"

"Yes." I murmured, tears stinging my eyes. "Yes."

I felt him shudder. And a deluge of hot semen rained down my back and trickled down my still burning bum.

He walked away, leaving me there, bent over, covered in his jizz, my cunt still wet and aching for him.

I cried. At that moment, I knew. He broke me. And I've never felt more alive.

www.ingramcontent.com/pod-product-compliance
Lightning Source LLC
LaVergne TN
LVHW010334200726
843507LV00010B/1484